Unlock Quantum Growth
Elevate Your Life

THE FREQUENCY EFFECT

A Life-Changing Guide to
Manifesting Brilliance and
Thriving Through Your Wildest Seasons

Angèle Lamothe

❅ LUCKY BOOK PUBLISHING

❖ LUCKY BOOK PUBLISHING

To request permissions, contact the publisher at hello@luckybookpublishing.com.

For speaking opportunities and coaching inquiries, visit www.angelelamothecoaching.com.

Paperback ISBN: 978-1-997775-39-3
Hardcover ISBN: 978-1-997775-40-9
E-book ISBN: 978-1-997775-38-6

First edition, November 2025

MY GIFT TO YOU

I am so glad you're here!

As my gift to you, enjoy FREE access to the audiobook
The Frequency Effect!

Simply scan the QR code below or visit
angelelamothecoaching.com to find out when
it will be available for free download.

ADVANCE PRAISE

More than a guide, it's a roadmap!

"*The Frequency Effect* is a roadmap to the beautiful life that awaits you. Angèle Lamothe has walked through the fire and emerged with wisdom, gratitude, and true awakening. As you read, you'll find yourself nodding, smiling, and whispering YES... exactly... Thank you. No matter where you are on your journey, this book will meet you there. Gently guiding you back to the truth of who you are and helping you awaken the magic that has always been within you."

– **Rich Sirop,** Mindset & Wellness Coach / Former Who Wants To Be A Millionaire Producer.

A blueprint to design the life you want!

"If you're ready to stop reacting to life and start designing it, this book is your blueprint. Through radical responsibility, gratitude, and energy mastery, *The Frequency Effect* empowers you to LEAD YOUR LIFE FROM THE INSIDE OUT, CLAIM your power, turn challenges into momentum, and accelerate personal and professional transformation."

An awesome guide to personal growth!

An entranceway to new visions and more authentic ways of being.

"Angèle Lamothe graciously holds the door for us. Ms. Lamothe is profoundly and intimately knowledgeable about her topic. As we learn from her book, she has been tried by life and her deep insights and rich wisdom have been annealed in the fires of experience. She is also a most congenial and gifted storyteller who interweaves the hard-won lessons she has learned in very positive ways into the fabric of her teaching. You will experience life and respond to it differently after reading *The Frequency Effect*. I couldn't put it down. Odds are, you won't be able to either."

> – **Bill Good,** #1 Best-Selling Author, TEDx Speaker, Teacher and Creator of The Good Factor Life.

Healing, practical and uplifting!

The Frequency Effect is a beautiful reminder that real transformation doesn't come from chasing more—it comes from tuning in. This book is a powerful invitation to reclaim your energy, align with your truth, and live with deep intention. As a physician, I've seen what happens when people disconnect from themselves and from their health. But I've also seen the profound healing that takes place when we pause, shift inward, and choose presence. This book is both a compass and a catalyst for that shift.

What I love most is how grounded it is in practice—not just theory. It teaches that change happens not in giant leaps, but in subtle shifts in how we show up every day. The emphasis on energy mastery, gratitude, and radical responsibility mirrors what I've seen in the health space: when people own their frequency, they own their future.

If you're ready to stop living on autopilot and start creating with intention, this book will meet you exactly where you are—and gently lift you higher. A true guide for living in alignment and wholeness."

    – **Dr. Kwadwo Kyeremanteng,** Physician, Key-Note Speaker, Best-Selling Author of "Prevention Over Prescription".

What an inspiring read!

"Angèle truly captured beautifully, what it means to align with your true power. Just like her, this book is full of passion and authenticity, leaving me truly touched by her stories and her message. If you ever have the chance to meet her in person, you will see how much of a gift she is and the energy she emits out with everyone she encounters. If you want to raise your frequency to a level that you may have only dreamed of, "*The Frequency Effect*" is the right place to start your journey."

> – **Ellie Laliberté.** Award winning Author of the book "Letters From You to You".

Angèle's presence shines through every chapter

"Compassionate, courageous, and wildly insightful. This book feels like sitting down with a trusted guide who fully believes in what's possible for you. *The Frequency Effect* is the kind of treasure you keep on your nightstand, highlight until the pages glow, and reach for every time you need to remember your own magic".

> – **Dr. Deonne Johnson,** Transformational Coach and Author of "From Tired to Inspired".

Very transformative!

"This book spoke to every cell of my body-radiant, practical, and deeply transformative. A masterclass in energy, alignment, and thriving. I am going to read and read this book a number of times. Highly and genuinely inspiring."

> – **Shelley A. Murdock,** Longevity & Strength Coach, Author of HEALTHY & FIT FOR LIFE and IN SEARCH OF LONGEVITY.

The Frequency Effect is both mirror and map

"A sacred synthesis of energy, embodiment, and evolution. Angèle Lamothe writes with the grace of a woman who has lived every word she teaches. She turns transformation into tangible practice, showing how alignment, truth, and radical responsibility become the architecture of an extraordinary life. This book is not about chasing higher vibrations — it's about stabilizing them. Frequency translated into form, power rooted in presence, and leadership lived as love in motion."

> – **Nadia S Krauss,** Author of "From Dreaming to Done: A Soul Map For What You Were Born to Do."

Real and relatable!

"*The Frequency Effect* is pure inspiration. Angèle Lamothe turns complex ideas about energy and growth into something real and relatable. Her words feel electric and full of heart, reminding you that alignment, not effort, is the key to change. Every chapter feels like a gentle wake-up call to your own power. It's the perfect mix of science, soul, and practical magic. If you're ready to raise your energy and create a life that actually feels good, this book is it."

– **Jenn Noble,** PCC Relationship Coach, TEDx Speaker, Podcast Host and Best Selling Author of "Dance of Attachment."

The perfect read to rise higher!

The Frequency Effect is a lovely recalibration for the soul. Angèle beautifully bridges energy and intention, science and spirit, showing us that real growth doesn't come from pushing harder but from aligning higher. Her words remind us that when we rise in frequency, we rise in life!

– **Julee Sung,** Global Consultant, Coach and Bestselling Author of "Thrive and SHINE."

ACKNOWLEDGEMENTS

I am deeply grateful for this life, for the gift of waking up each day, for the moments that shape me, and for the incredible souls who have crossed my path. Every person, every experience, every challenge has carried meaning and purpose, even when I couldn't see it at the time.

You may never know how much you've touched me and my family. Your love, support, and presence, in big and small ways, have left a lasting mark on our hearts. Never underestimate the power of generosity or the difference you can make in someone's life. What feels small to you may mean the world to someone else. When you give with sincerity and love, it expands far beyond what you can see.

I'm forever grateful for every person I've met and every lesson along the way. Life has taught me that what truly matters isn't what we have but how we show up, with kindness, gratitude, and authenticity.

To my three incredible children, Émerick, Cédric, and Christophe, thank you for teaching me how to love without limits. To my parents, my greatest supporters and guiding posts, thank you for your endless belief in me. To my sisters, soul sisters, close colleagues, and dear and closest friends, I'm so grateful for the laughter, the tears, and the unwavering bond that holds us forever.

Life continues to remind me that love is what endures. Every moment shared, every act of care, every bit of kindness and love lives on, and for that, I am eternally grateful.

Angèle xo

MY DREAM

My mission is to ignite a global awakening: to empower over 5 million people to rise, reclaim their energy, and live in full alignment with their extraordinary potential. This is more than a vision; it's a movement. It's about owning your frequency, elevating your impact, and becoming the light that inspires others to expand with you.

The Frequency Effect was born from the depths of my own transformation, from walking through my son's health challenges to discovering the power of presence, resilience, and energetic mastery. It's shaped by years of guiding hundreds of individuals to activate their greatness, expand their energy, and live with clarity and purpose.

Over the next two years, I am committed to amplifying this message globally, speaking on 50 stages or more, appearing on at least 100 podcasts, and sharing this mission as an international bestselling author.

This book is not just my story. It's our collective

call to rise. It's a guide, a mirror, and a catalyst for transformation. It reminds you that the life you desire isn't somewhere "out there," it's already within reach, waiting for your alignment, your awareness, your choice.

The Frequency Effect is more than something you read. It's something you embody. It's a declaration that now is your time to rise, to lead from your energy, to live your truth, and to become the light that awakens others to their own power.

Everything in this universe is energy, and you are transmitting a frequency in every moment. Every thought you think, every word you speak, every act of kindness you offer sends a signal into the world, a frequency that shapes reality. This book is a reminder of your power, your freedom, and your infinite potential. You are not waiting for permission, and you are not here to carry the world. When you take ownership of your thoughts, emotions, and actions, you become the catalyst for extraordinary transformation. You are here to take radical responsibility for your own energy, your own happiness, your own choices. True change begins within you, and as you rise, you inspire others to rise with you. That's where real quantum change begins.

And because change must ripple outward, 30% of

all proceeds from this book will go directly to mental health access and various transformative causes.

The world is shifting, and amidst the noise and uncertainty, your light matters now more than ever. Every thought you hold, every word you speak, and every act of kindness you partake in creates a ripple that reaches farther than you can imagine. Together, we rise, elevating ourselves, our communities, and the collective consciousness of the world.

INTRODUCTION

Everything in this universe is energy, flowing, vibrating, responding. Whether you realize it or not, you are always transmitting a frequency. Every thought, every belief, every word, every action sends out a signal, and life faithfully mirrors it back.

I didn't realize it at the time, but I had been living in the noise of the world, shaped by societal expectations, outdated paradigms, and beliefs about what success should look like. I pushed harder, sacrificed more, and measured myself against someone else's standards. On the outside, it appeared like progress; inside, I felt drained, restless, and disconnected.

The truth is, nothing was wrong with me. I was simply out of alignment with my own energy and had been tuning to the wrong frequency. Recognizing this changed everything. The restlessness became a signal to reconnect with my own rhythm, to live by my own standards, and to define success on my terms. That choice to tune into myself instead of the noise was the first step toward true fulfillment and growth.

And here is the deep truth that shifts everything: It doesn't have to be complicated. It doesn't have to be overwhelming. Transformation happens step by step, moment by moment. With each small choice, you begin to align with higher frequencies. With each conscious breath, you anchor into your power. With each intentional shift, you open the door to more ease, more flow, more time, and more abundance. The extraordinary life you crave isn't built overnight; it is created in the simple, repeatable practices that elevate your energy and expand your reality.

It's born from the lessons we carry, from growth and wisdom acquired through hardships, and through the gratitude of choice. The Frequency Effect is not about slowing down your ambition. It's about amplifying your impact by mastering your energy, expanding wider, and shifting your frequency so radically that your external reality cannot help but shift to match your inner transformation. This is not about more effort; it is about more alignment. Not about more force, but about more flow.

That's who you've always been, limitless, divine, and far more powerful than you've been led to believe

Throughout this book, you'll learn how to:

- Take Radical Responsibility: Stop giving your power away; own your growth, choices, and energy.

- Elevate Your Energy: Convert stress, fear, and chaos into flow, abundance, and joy.

- Shift Your Vibration: See obstacles as invitations, challenges as catalysts, and setbacks as momentum.

- Gratitude Growth: Reframe challenges, expand perspective, and amplify results.

- Magnetize Opportunities: Attract people, experiences, and situations that resonate with your vision.

- Gain Clarity & Focus: Navigate overwhelm with intention, vision, and aligned action.

- Quantum Leap: Thrive in your life by creating power, and a legacy of impact.

The doorway is open, and the moment is now. This is your invitation to step boldly into the next level of your life. To claim your power. To reclaim your energy. To rise beyond limitation. To thrive. To transform. Every obstacle is an initiation into greater strength. Every resistance is a call back into alignment. Every challenge carries within it the seed of your next quantum leap.

You are the common denominator of your life, which means you are also the key. The power to unlock your extraordinary life has always been in your hands. Every breath you take and every choice you make is an opportunity to pivot, expand, and rise higher than you ever imagined.

This book is not just information, it's your reclamation. Your road map back to the limitless power and truth of who you really are. And as you uncover yourself, step by step, moment by moment, you will open the doorway to more time, more abundance, more freedom, and more joy than you've ever experienced before. Your next level isn't waiting for you to work harder; it's waiting for you to tune into the Frequency Effect. Because when you align with that frequency, you don't just transform your own life, you create ripples that elevate everyone around you. When you step into your power, you become a catalyst for change, activating collective transformation and drawing into your field exactly what matches your elevated state.

CONTENTS

SECTION ONE
THE GREAT QUANTUM SHIFT

The courage to see your blind spots is one key to your quantum leaps.

The Great Shift begins the moment you choose to stop looking away or blaming, and start looking within. It takes radical courage to face the parts of yourself you've avoided, the stories you've inherited, and the layers of illusion you've carried for too long. But every layer you peel back is a doorway, elevating your frequency, unlocking clarity, and revealing the truth of who you really are. When you meet this process with gratitude, the universe responds, guiding you to the very blind spots that once held you back. The universe holds a mirror to your blind spots, and the faster you're willing to see them, the faster you rise, stepping into alignment and power, with the highest, unstoppable version of yourself. This is where transformation becomes exponential. This is **The Great Quantum Shift**.

CHAPTER 1
THE GREAT REMEMBERING: SHEDDING LAYERS OF LIMITING BELIEFS

"In the process of letting go, you will lose many things from the past, but you will find yourself."
— Deepak Chopra

Layers That Were Never Mine: Reclaim Your Power

I spent a big part of my life shrinking. I adapted, softened, and dimmed myself to fit into spaces that weren't built for me. I gave more than I had, compromised endlessly, and measured my worth by how much I could do for others. I thought that was how to stay safe, to be loved, to belong. But it didn't work. It never worked. Every compromise I made, every time I silenced my own needs, only buried me deeper under expectations and beliefs that were never mine to begin with. I lost my voice, my power, my energy, and for years, I thought that meant something was wrong with me.

I wasn't broken. I was misaligned. I was living by someone else's rules, carrying burdens I never agreed to, following patterns that kept me small. I now see that the universe was never punishing me; it was waiting for me to reclaim my power. Every setback, every challenge, every resistance an invitation to rise, not a signal that I had failed.

I began to notice how much energy I had been giving away. How much of myself I had surrendered to rules, expectations, and inherited stories. Every "yes" that wasn't mine, every fear I absorbed from others, every compromise I made to feel safe, had cost me time, clarity, and power. The truth hit hard: The life I wanted, the impact I was capable of, and the freedom I craved had always been mine to claim, but I had been standing in my own way.

The universe had always been present, responding, guiding, and offering its wisdom. The energy, clarity, and power I sought were never missing. They were always there; I just had to quiet the noise, release the distractions, and stop shrinking in order to access them. Every layer I shed, every pattern I released, every truth I embraced restored my authority, expanded my influence, and strengthened my presence. I was no longer waiting, no longer shrinking; I was stepping fully into the power that was my birthright.

Transformation does not require force or perfection. It begins with awareness, honesty, and alignment with truth. Every conscious step compounds. The layers I carried were never mine to begin with. They were inherited fears, collective conditioning, and the weight of generations before me.

The Weight of Forgotten Truth

I began shedding the layers, one by one. And let me be clear, shedding is not glamorous or easy. It's uncomfortable, sometimes painfully lonely, and it forces you to confront parts of yourself you've kept hidden, even from your own awareness. It demands that you face the truth, question the stories that have shaped your identity, and release versions of yourself that no longer serve your life. It tests your courage, your values, and your willingness to stand fully in your own power. But it is necessary and absolutely worth it, because on the other side of release is real freedom, the freedom to create a life aligned with your extraordinary truth, not dictated by the expectations of others, a life that has always been waiting for you.

I learned that you cannot rise into higher frequencies while holding onto the old ones. You cannot claim your power while dimming your light for the comfort of others. Every "yes" that isn't yours, every compromise made from fear, obligation, or guilt, every moment you shrink to avoid judgment, all of it keeps you anchored to lower energies. Fear, shame, and doubt create invisible chains that bind you to a version of yourself that was never meant to last. True alignment requires release. True growth demands honesty.

I started asking myself the hard questions: What layers am I carrying that were never mine? What inherited beliefs no longer serve me? What would my life look like if I stopped dimming my light for the comfort of others?

As I began shedding, I felt the weight I had been carrying, of beliefs, fears, and expectations that didn't belong to me. I recognized how often I had given away my power in small, nearly invisible ways: saying yes when I meant no, staying silent when truth was required, pretending to be fine when I was not. Each act of self-abandonment built another layer, another barrier between who I was and who I came here to be. With every layer removed, I reclaimed a piece of my power, a piece of my clarity, and a piece of the extraordinary life that was always within reach.

The real work begins when you are willing to see those patterns through the eyes of love, not judgment. When you can look at your life, your relationships, your habits, and your choices with compassion and honesty. Healing doesn't come from rejection; it comes from recognition. You meet each layer not with shame, but with grace. You begin to understand that every pattern, every defense, was once a form of protection. And the moment you see it clearly, you can thank it, bless it, and release it.

That is the essence of the *unlayering*: not destruction, but remembrance. Not punishment, but liberation. The more truth you allow, the lighter you become and the higher you elevate.

When Love Changes Shape

For me, it started in my marriage, with small, quiet acts of defiance that were really acts of returning to myself. For years, I had been too quiet, too polite, too willing to shrink to make others comfortable. I said yes when I wanted to say no. I smiled when I was exhausted. I gave everything when I was empty. I silenced my voice to keep the peace, believing that was love, believing that was loyalty, believing that was just how life was meant to be. But inside, I was running on empty. I ignored the emptiness. I rationalized it. I apologized for it. I minimized it.

Still, the whisper inside me refused to go away. Over time, it grew louder, echoing through sleepless nights, insisting that I could no longer ignore it. It wasn't chaos that woke me. It was the truth.

For years, I had trained everyone around me how to treat me. I had shown that my needs came last, that my silence was acceptable, and that my worth was measured by how much I could give. So when I finally changed the rules, when I started saying no, setting boundaries, speaking my truth, it was no surprise that the ripples shook everything around me. I felt the pushback, the judgment, the discomfort of those accustomed to my compliance.

But I could not blame anyone. There was no betrayal, no explosive ending, no villain. The unraveling of my marriage was not the result of a single act; it was the consequence of years of slow depletion. Two people giving from empty cups, both trying to hold everything together without realizing that love cannot thrive where truth is silenced. I had believed that, if I gave more, loved harder, sacrificed deeper, it would be enough. But in giving everything away, I lost myself. I gave away my power. Over time, it drained the life from me, leaving me hollow, invisible, and desperate to reclaim what was always mine.

The Cost of Shrinking

Motherhood has been one of the greatest joys of my life, and also one of the most demanding responsibilities. My children became my anchor, my reason, my heart. But somewhere along the way, I disappeared inside that role. My needs became negotiable. My dreams were postponed until "someday." My desires felt selfish, luxuries I hadn't earned. I believed that giving until I was empty was proof of love, that exhaustion was the price of being a good mother and partner. But over time, I realized my children didn't need a mother who was always available. They needed a mother who was fully alive. A woman lit from within, who embodied what it means to live truthfully and completely. That realization terrified me, because admitting it demanded change. Change meant disruption. It meant confronting the truth that my happiness, my wholeness, and my energy were not optional; they were essential.

Sleepless Nights and Self-Doubt

The nights were the hardest. When the house was quiet, I would lie awake, my mind racing with questions I was too afraid to voice. Was I selfish for wanting more? Was I betraying my vows? Would my children resent me for choosing myself? Would

I regret this later? The weight of these questions pressed down, fueled by the voices of expectation: a "good woman" stays, a "good wife" endures, a "good mother" sacrifices herself to keep everyone else whole.

But beneath that pressure, another voice persisted. Steady. Clear. It reminded me that I wasn't running from anything. I was returning to myself. To my voice. To my alignment. To my power. That realization changed everything. I understood that love doesn't always stay the same. It can evolve, shift, and take new forms without being wrong. The truth I had ignored in my marriage, the misalignments, the frustrations, the compromises, was not failure; it was evidence of growth and change. I had once believed that giving everything guaranteed permanence, but I learned that love doesn't always work that way. It isn't about holding on at any cost or sacrificing until nothing remains. Sometimes, even after you've given your best, love changes, and acceptance is necessary.

In the aftermath, I chose gratitude. Gratitude for the love we shared, the life we built, and the three children who are the center of our story. Gratitude for the lessons that came from discomfort and pain, which strengthened me and deepened my understanding. Gratitude for the ending itself, because it created space for alignment, authenticity, and freedom. My ending was quiet and deliberate. There was no drama, no betrayal, no sudden collapse, only clarity. The disconnection unfolded gradually, day by day, until I could no longer ignore it. I realized I could love fully while still choosing myself. Awakening didn't require chaos; alignment, truth, and self-respect were enough. I didn't need anyone's approval to act with integrity.

Reclaiming Your Life and Energy—Own Your Truth and Shape Your World

Forgiveness invites you to release what no longer belongs to you. It asks you to look at where you may still be carrying resentment, blame, or regret, and to consider how those emotions might be keeping you anchored in the past. What would change if you forgave yourself for the times you stayed silent or small? What peace might you feel if you forgave others not because they were right, but because you deserve to be free?

Taking full responsibility for your life means reclaiming your power. It means asking yourself where you've been waiting for someone else to change before you do, and what parts of your story you've outgrown. Are you ready to let go of old labels, pleaser, fixer, perfectionist, and step into the fullness of who you are becoming? Each day offers you a new opportunity to decide how you will show up, what energy you will bring, and the kind of impact you want to create.

Living in alignment calls you back to your truth. It's an invitation to notice where your actions don't yet match your values, and where you may still be performing instead of being. What would it look like to make choices that reflect your deepest priorities, not your fears or obligations? What shifts could you make today to live more deliberately, with intention and authenticity?

Growth begins when you stop resisting change and start learning from it. Life keeps presenting lessons until you integrate them. What is the current season of your life teaching you? Where are you still surviving instead of expanding? Transformation doesn't come from what happens to you, it comes from how you respond, how you rise, and how you allow awareness to move you forward.

All types of love evolve, romantic, platonic, familial, and even the love we have for ourselves. It doesn't always disappear, sometimes it simply changes form. Can you honor what has ended while staying open to what's next? Can you allow love to express itself through understanding, freedom, and compassion instead of control or fear? Every ending, whether in a relationship, friendship, or season of life, creates space for something new to emerge. Every moment of acceptance becomes a bridge to greater clarity, connection, and peace.

As you continue to grow, you might ask yourself: What energy do I want to bring into the world? What truth am I ready to live out loud? What legacy of authenticity and courage do I want to leave behind? Your life is not defined by the past, but by the choices you make now—the choices that align you with who you truly are and what you are here to create.

Releasing what no longer serves you is not losing but discovering the truth of who you are beneath the roles, fears, and expectations that once controlled your life. Fear is a signal that tells you that growth is available, that stepping forward requires courage, and that what lies ahead demands action. Letting go isn't loss, it's an energetic upgrade. In that upgrade, you create space to welcome the new.

I've learned that we are the authors of our lives. If you don't consciously write your story, someone else will. Every decision, every boundary, every truth you honor becomes a sentence in the narrative you're creating. Living intentionally, aligned with your values, guided by your truth, and anchored in self-awareness, is the highest expression of self-respect. It's how you reclaim your power, direct the course of your life, and define the impact and legacy you want to leave behind.

Reflection Exercises

Take a journal and spend some time with the following prompts:

- Where am I giving away my energy, influence, or authority? What choices have I made to please others instead of honoring myself?

- Which beliefs that I've inherited no longer serve me? Where in my life am I living by someone else's rules or expectations?

- What fear is keeping me from taking the next step in my life? If I acted without self-doubt, what would I attempt today?

- How does my energy affect the people and environments around me?

- Where can I raise my frequency to create greater influence and alignment?

- What would it look like to fully express myself without apology?

- Which compromises have I made that I can now release?

Affirmations

I am fully in command of my life.
I release everything that holds
me back. I claim my power, my
freedom, and my truth without
hesitation. I act boldly, choose
fiercely, and create my reality with
clarity and purpose. I will no longer
wait. I will no longer settle. I rise
into my full potential now.

CHAPTER 2
THE COMPASS ALWAYS POINTS INWARD: STOP OUTSOURCING YOUR WORTH

"At the center of your being you have the answer; you know who you are and you know what you want." — Lao Tzu

---

Owning Your Value—When Worth Meets Boundaries

This chapter is about reclaiming your inner authority, returning to your truth, and trusting the divine guidance that has always been within you. The quiet inner knowing that is more powerful and reliable than any external measure of success or validation. It's about stopping the outsourcing of your value and stepping fully into the life you were meant to live.

Self-worth isn't given. Worth isn't earned. Worth is claimed. It begins with one unwavering choice: *I am enough. I deserve to be happy. I decide how worthy I am.*

Worth is internal. It cannot be negotiated, taken, or granted by others. When you stop outsourcing your worth, you stop negotiating your identity. When you turn inward, you discover a foundation that no circumstance, situation, or person can shake. When you trust your inner compass, even the scariest and darkest paths feel aligned and exactly where you are meant to be because the universe is always guiding you towards it!

Boundaries as Energy Protection

When we enter relationships, whether romantic, familial, friendly, or professional, we often carry unconscious beliefs about what makes us valuable. These beliefs shape how we give, receive, and connect. Many of us learned early that love, approval, and belonging were conditional. I did too.

Some of the stories that guided my behavior sounded like this:

- *If you work hard at love, it will last; divorce is failure.*

- *Leaving a relationship is selfish, even if you no longer feel love*

- *It's wrong to outgrow friends, even when the friendship no longer supports you.*

- *Friendship means putting your needs second.*

- *Being needed means being loved.*

- *Boundaries hurt people; saying no is rejection.*

These ideas became my inner rules. Over time, I started equating being needed with being worthy. The more others depended on me, the more valuable I felt. My sense of worth became tied to how well I could meet others' expectations. When people were happy with me, I felt secure. When they were disappointed, I felt guilt and tried harder to prove my value.

Eventually, I realized this pattern wasn't about love. It was about external validation. My energy was constantly focused outward, trying to earn acceptance instead of honoring alignment. Through these experiences, the universe was providing feedback. Every imbalance, every emotional drain, was a signal to look at where I was giving my power away. The more I noticed, the more I requested universal guidance and the faster I quantum leaped change and embodied these new ways of being.

The shift came when I began to see relationships as mirrors for growth. Instead of asking, "How can I make this work for others?" I started asking, "What is this teaching me about my own boundaries, needs, and values?" This awareness changed everything. I started to understand that my worth was never something to earn. It wasn't tied to being needed, liked, or approved of. It was always there, steady and whole, waiting for me to recognize it. I began to see that real love and connection grow when honesty and boundaries are present, not when I silence myself to keep others comfortable. Discomfort in relationships no longer felt like failure; it became feedback, a signal showing me where I was meant to grow next. I realized that alignment creates authentic connection, and the people who truly value me will adjust to truth, not performance.

When I began living from that awareness, everything around me started to shift. The relationships built on dependency quietly fell away, and the ones rooted in mutual respect and authenticity deepened. I no longer needed to prove my value. I could just be. And in that space of being, I noticed how differently life responded. The more I honored my truth, the more aligned experiences and people entered my life.

I'm grateful for what these lessons revealed. Every challenge, ending, and uncomfortable moment became a quiet teacher. Each one showed me where I was ready to grow, where I was still playing small, and where a different choice could open a new direction.

I began to understand that life always mirrors our inner world. The way I thought, spoke, and showed up shaped the frequency I lived in, and that frequency became the foundation for everything I experienced. When I started to choose honesty over avoidance, gratitude over resistance, and alignment over obligation, my reality began to shift. People, opportunities, and outcomes started matching the energy I was cultivating within.

Living this way has become both a discipline and a devotion. It requires courage to see yourself clearly and to act from that awareness, even when it means letting go. It also asks for trust, that what ends is not punishment, but preparation. That space is being cleared for something that reflects your growth.

With time, I learned to see every experience as guidance. The moments I resisted most were often the ones that revealed my next level of strength, boundaries, or clarity. The more I stayed honest with myself, the more supported I felt by life itself.

If you find yourself in a season of change, pause and ask: *What is this moment trying to show me? What is it asking me to release or embody?*

Each time you respond with awareness instead of fear, you raise your energy. You step closer to peace. You become the steady force behind the life you are creating.

Ask yourself where your value depends on others' approval. Think of a decision you avoided or delayed because of others' expectations. *If I acted from my own authority and worth, what would I choose?*

Boundaries, Energy, and the Cost of Overgiving

I had spent years trying to earn love, as it's easy to mistake external validation for safety. But the universe is always communicating through energy, showing us where we are aligned and where we are not. The exhaustion, resentment, and emptiness I felt after overgiving were not signs of failure but gifts guiding me back home to myself.

I realized that the universe had been whispering to me all along through these moments of discomfort. Every time I ignored my limits, silenced my truth, or said yes when I meant no, I was being gently redirected to pause, listen, and realign. The guidance was never missing; I was just too busy seeking approval to hear it.

True worth isn't measured by how much we give or how needed we are, it's measured by the energy and intention behind our actions. When we act from alignment instead of fear, our energy expands, and life responds in kind. Scarcity attracts more scarcity; worthiness attracts opportunities, relationships, and experiences that reflect our value.

The shift happens when you trust that your value doesn't need proving. Listen to your inner guidance, those subtle nudges, sensations, and feelings of expansion or contraction. They are universal intelligence speaking through you. Feeling drained or off-center isn't a flaw; it's feedback and a beautiful opportunity to return to alignment.

Every time you honor your truth over fear, you claim your power. Saying no to what depletes you is saying yes to yourself. Boundaries are self-respect, and alignment is magnetic. The universe mirrors the energy you emit, trust it, follow it, and life flows effortlessly in your favor.

Ask yourself: How does the universe speak to you, through intuition, emotions, repetition, or physical sensations? What unfolds when you actually follow its guidance?

Letting Go and Turning Inward

Walking away from relationships, friendships, and situations that no longer serve you is never easy. It can be messy, emotional, and uncertain, and still, it is one of the most powerful and freeing acts of self-honor. Letting go creates the space and energy for what is truly meant for you to enter. It's not about erasing the past but acknowledging it with grace, love, and gratitude, for the connection, the memories, the growth, and the version of you that learned through it all. Society may call it selfish, but I've learned that following your inner compass is the most self-respecting and life-affirming choice you can make.

I have come to understand that every choice to step away from what no longer serves me is not a loss but an act of alignment and claiming my own power. I am choosing myself, my priorities, my life, and my truth. I have learned to release guilt and to meet discomfort, endings, and uncertainty with awareness and gratitude. Gratitude has become the highest frequency I can hold, and I have seen how the energy I carry shapes everything I attract. Most of my life is spent in the thoughts and feelings I nurture, and when I do so intentionally, growth and opportunity follow naturally, almost effortlessly. I can honor my past, every person and experience that has shaped me, without attachment or regret, while stepping fully into the future I am building. Gratitude is the frequency that unlocks quantum change, that turns pain into wisdom and endings into new beginnings, while honoring the past.

Through this process, I started living more intentionally. I no longer measured my worth by how much I gave or how much I was needed, but by how deeply I honored my truth. I replaced approval-seeking with self-trust and people-pleasing with alignment. I learned that my energy teaches others how to treat me, especially my children. By choosing authenticity, I show them that boundaries are healthy, that self-worth is non-negotiable, and that love grounded in truth is the most powerful kind.

The messiness is still real. There are moments of doubt, grief, and vulnerability. But now I see that part of the journey as sacred too. Growth doesn't have to look perfect to be beautiful. The tears, the letting go, the uncertainty, all of it is proof of courage, of choosing to rise instead of remain.

Each time I honor myself, I rise a little higher. Each time I choose gratitude over fear, I align a little deeper with the life I'm meant to live. The universe meets that energy every time, matching it with opportunities, clarity, and connection that reflect my highest vibration. This is what freedom feels like, not because everything is perfect, but because I'm finally aligned with my truth. Your worth doesn't need validation. It needs alignment. What decisions in your life are being driven by fear rather than truth?

Energy Awareness and Embodying Worth

The compass always points inward, not to the noise of others' expectations, but to the quiet wisdom of your soul. True worth cannot be earned, only remembered. It isn't built through overgiving or performing to feel loved. When I stopped trying to earn validation, everything began to shift. The truth is, no matter how much time I spent trying to control other people's perceptions of me, it was impossible, and attempting it drained my energy and diminished my power.

What we can control are our thoughts, actions, and beliefs. When we focus on these, we reclaim our energy and create a frequency that aligns with our highest self. By choosing to act from truth rather than fear, we stop giving from emptiness and begin giving from fullness. We stop chasing approval and begin attracting relationships, opportunities, and experiences that reflect our authentic worth. The more consistently we honor our inner compass, the more the universe mirrors back the energy we hold, showing us what supports our growth and what no longer serves us.

Each conscious choice to align with our truth

strengthens our sense of value, raises our vibration, and opens the door to abundance, clarity, and meaningful connection. True power comes from within, and when we operate from that place, everything around us begins to reflect it.

I began asking myself important questions and reframing my beliefs:

- *Am I honoring my truth or someone else's expectation?*

- *Is this choice coming from fear or alignment?*

- *Does this support my energy, joy, and growth?*

- *Am I showing love from fullness rather than obligation?*

- *Am I choosing relationships that lift and honor me?*

These questions became a guide for reclaiming my power. When worth lives inside, no rejection, disappointment, or loss can diminish it. You stop chasing love and begin attracting it. You stop giving from emptiness and begin giving from a full cup. I affirm: *I am valuable and worthy because I choose it.*

I began tracking my energy carefully. Before saying yes, I asked myself: Do I want to do this, or am I acting from fear? Even when I desire to help, do I have the capacity right now, and is this aligned with my vision and truth? I tuned into my energy: Does this choice energize or drain me? I practiced small boundaries: pauses, silence, and discomfort allowed to exist long enough to make choices from clarity rather than impulse.

Each morning, I meditated, set intentions, and asked the universe for guidance and growth. Over time, I realized that self-worth comes from keeping promises to yourself, not from meeting everyone else's expectations. Choosing honesty and allowing others to feel disappointment became an act of self-respect, not selfishness. I am not responsible for how another person might be feeling. This feeling belongs to them and them only.

I noticed how much energy I had spent trying to control outcomes: other people's opinions, work results, timing. Control created tension and false security. I shifted my focus to what I truly have power over: my attention, my joy, my alignment, and my sense of worth.

I stopped holding every piece together and focused on how I showed up, what I believed, and where I placed my energy. Choosing myself became sacred. I am grateful for every lesson, every relationship, and every challenge that showed me where I needed to grow. I thank the universe for guiding me back to myself, for revealing the opportunities to expand, and for teaching me that living from alignment and authenticity attracts more of what supports my highest good. Each conscious choice strengthens my energy, raises my frequency, and opens the door to deeper growth, richer experiences, and relationships that honor the truth of who I am.

You don't attract what you want; you attract what you are. How are your daily choices reflecting the level of worth you want to embody?

Living in Alignment with Your Worth

Worth is reinforced through choice. Every decision, what you allow, what you agree to, and how you speak to yourself, either builds or weakens your sense of value. I began pausing before reacting and asking three questions: Does this support my energy or drain it? Am I acting from alignment or seeking approval? Who am I becoming by choosing this? That pause changed everything. It helped me make decisions that protected my energy, respected my limits, and reflected my priorities.

When you begin choosing from awareness rather than habit, your energy shifts. You stop overextending for approval and start creating space for what genuinely supports you. The energy you release into the world mirrors what you hold within. When your choices are grounded in self-respect, you naturally attract people and opportunities that match that level of respect. You no longer chase validation or outcomes but align with them through your behavior, presence, and boundaries.

Your worth doesn't grow by doing more; it grows by honoring your energy and attention. Every yes that feels right strengthens self-trust. Every no that protects your peace reinforces self-respect. Over time, the quality of your energy determines the quality of what you draw in. You don't need to prove your value when you live it through conscious decisions that reflect who you truly are and what you stand for. You are the only one who can define your worth, and people will match it and treat you accordingly, so own it, all of it!

Your worth isn't proven. It's lived. Each time you choose presence over people-pleasing, truth over performance, and calm over control, you reclaim it. Worth was never lost. It was waiting for you to remember who decides.

You don't attract what you want. You attract what you are.

Worth isn't earned through effort; it's expressed

through alignment.

How can you live your worth more intentionally in your choices, your energy, and your boundaries, today?

Leaping into Defining My Worth

There are moments that don't just change your path but the trajectory of your life forever. This was one of those moments. I'll never forget the day my friend called. It wasn't just a phone call; it was an invitation to step into a version of myself I hadn't yet met but knew existed. On one side stood safety, predictability, and the illusion of control. On the other side waited growth, expansion, and the life I was ready to claim. She told me about a leadership program that had completely transformed her life. I could see it in her energy, in her confidence, and in the way her life had shifted dramatically. As I listened, my stomach tightened. It sounded bold. It sounded unfamiliar. It sounded terrifying.

At that time, I had just gone through my divorce and was carefully saving money for furniture, for a couch, a table, the pieces that would make my house feel like home again. Those savings represented stability for my kids. But suddenly, it was being called to a higher purpose: invest in furniture or invest in myself. My rational mind screamed with fear: What will people think? I don't even have a living room set yet. This isn't responsible. What if I fail? What if the money never comes back? These thoughts were fear masquerading as logic, scarcity disguised as practicality.

Beneath the fear, though, was a quieter, unwavering voice: *This opportunity is here for a reason. Trust it. Stop overthinking. Surrender. Take the leap. The universe always meets you wherever you choose to grow.*

I chose to follow that voice. I asked myself the question that mattered most: *If I say yes, am I honoring my soul? Am I stepping into the woman I was created to become? What example am I setting for my children about what's possible and who defines worth?* The answer was instant and clear: YES. So I made the leap. I emptied my savings and enrolled in the program. On paper, it made no sense, but in my heart, it was perfect. I trusted the universe to take care of the rest.

And it did. The money came. The furniture came. The support came. Because the moment I said yes to my worth, the universe mirrored that energy back. That choice changed something inside of me, and I realized abundance is not about possessions; it's about belief in what you deserve. Worth is not measured by productivity, approval, or external validation. Worth is a vibration, a frequency, a declaration: *I trust life to support me because I am aligned with my truth and inherently worthy of abundance.*

I am grateful for that moment, for my friend's courage and vulnerability to share her journey, and for the lesson the universe presented. Every step, every fear, every decision to follow my inner guidance strengthened my energy, expanded my vision, and created space for more growth, opportunity, and aligned relationships. When your choices come from fear, life mirrors fear. When they come from self-trust, life mirrors expansion, abundance, and the unlimited possibilities available to those who step fully into their own worth.

Your value is not determined by possessions, titles, or other people's approval. It is a vibration and a frequency you embody. Fear often disguises itself as logic or scarcity. See it as a signal that growth is waiting on the other side.

Worth Is Internal, Not Conditional

The universe doesn't respond to your words. It responds to your energy. It mirrors the vibration of how you define your worth. That leap taught me one thing: I alone decide what I'm worthy of. The moment you stop measuring yourself by what's safe, reasonable, or acceptable, and instead align with your inner power, everything begins to shift. You stop chasing validation and start magnetizing opportunities that reflect your self-belief.

Gratitude became my anchor, not just for the easy moments, but for the fear too. Fear became proof that I was stretching beyond old limits. Every leap of faith turned into an act of gratitude, a signal to the universe: I am ready for more. Looking back, that phone call wasn't random. It was divinely timed, a soul-level invitation to stop living small and start living aligned.

Now, I pass that invitation to you. Where in your life are you waiting for permission? Which dreams are you rationalizing away because they feel too risky, too indulgent, too big? Which leaps terrify you precisely because, deep down, you know they will transform you? Stop seeking approval to become who you already are. Stop bargaining with your worth. The leap that scares you most is the one that will expand you most.

The universe is always listening. It responds not to what you want, but to what you believe you deserve. When you act from abundance instead of fear, when your choices come from self-trust instead of scarcity, life rises to meet your frequency. Ask yourself now: What leap is waiting for me, and when will I finally choose it? The answer is simple. The time is now. The universe is already waiting for your yes.

Reflection Exercises

Take a journal and spend some time with the following prompts:

- Where in your life are you outsourcing your worth to the opinions, approval, or acceptance of others?

- What would shift if you allowed your inner compass, not fear, expectation, or guilt, to guide your next step?

- What layers of guilt, shame, or attachment are you ready to shed in order to honor your truth?

- Which relationships, habits, or commitments consistently drain your energy?

- Where have you confused being needed with being loved?

- What truth have you been avoiding because you fear disappointing someone?

Affirmations

I am worthy. I always have been. My value is inherent and unshakable. I move with clarity, not fear. Every decision I make in alignment expands my power. The universe supports my every step. Abundance flows to me because I am aligned with truth. Saying no protects my peace. Saying yes honors my soul. I own my energy. I choose my boundaries. I define my worth. I am guided, powerful, and limitless.

CHAPTER 3
FROM GUILT TO FAME

"Some of us think holding on makes us strong, but sometimes it is letting go." — Eckhart Tolle

---

Turning Guilt and Fear into Freedom

For much of my life, guilt was my default state. It wasn't a passing emotion but the lens through which I experienced everything. I woke up in it, carried it through the day, and brought it to bed with me every night. I felt guilty for everything: for not being enough, for wanting more than what I had, for saying yes when my body screamed no, and for saying no when I was terrified of disappointing someone.

Beneath the guilt was shame. Shame whispered the questions I could never answer: *Who are you to want what you want? Who are you to shine? Why can't you just be grateful for what you already have?* These whispers became so constant that I mistook them for my own truth. I carried them, unaware they had been placed on me long before I was born, as the residue of collective trauma, inherited paradigms, and unspoken societal rules.

It took time, reflection, and courage to see that guilt is rarely truth. It is often inherited, passed down through lineages, cultures, and systems that conditioned us to doubt our own worth. And yet, as I peeled back the layers, I discovered something luminous beneath it all: my true essence, patiently waiting for me.

This chapter is about transformation, the alchemy of turning guilt into fuel, shame into courage, and fear into power. It is about moving from hiding in the shadows of *not enough* into standing fully visible in the light of *more than enough*. It is about remembering that your worth is inherent and non-negotiable, and that your life, energy, and presence are gifts to the world.

When I say "fame," I don't mean celebrity (though that may follow for anyone who chooses it), but rather becoming known to your own soul. It means embracing your full radiance, unapologetically choosing yourself, and stepping into freedom.

I am deeply grateful for every moment of guilt, every

moment of shame, and every fear that once held me back, because they became my teachers. I thank the universe for showing me exactly where I needed to grow, for guiding me to reclaim my power, and for mirroring back the energy I chose to cultivate. The more I aligned with my truth, the more the universe responded in kind, opening doors, opportunities, and connections that reflected the worth, courage, and abundance I was now embodying. Each lesson, each challenge, each relationship was a mirror of growth, and embracing them with gratitude allowed me to rise into the life I was always meant to live.

When you feel guilt, shame, or fear, what is it trying to show you about where you need to grow or realign? How can you transform that energy into fuel for courage, clarity, and empowerment?

The Whisper Beneath the Noise

When I began to question the guilt, another voice emerged. Unlike shame, this voice didn't scold. Unlike guilt, it didn't accuse. It whispered.

I discovered it first in meditation, a quiet hum beneath my breath. Then it revealed itself in journaling, spilling onto the page as words I didn't even know I carried. In stillness, it arrived as a subtle nudge, pointing me toward something unseen yet undeniably real. That voice, my intuition, my higher self had always been there, waiting, but I had ignored it for too long. Once I finally started making time throughout my day so that I could listen, it grew louder, clearer, stronger. And with it came courage. I began asking the questions I once found too bold, too esoteric, too much.

Universe, show me the way.

Bring me the people who can guide me.

Reveal everything I can't yet see.

Awaken me to the possibilities I have forgotten.

And slowly, life began to answer.

What if guilt isn't the voice of truth, but the echo of old conditioning?

The Breaking Point

One of the hardest seasons of my life was during my divorce, yet it was also one of the most expansive. I will never forget the night I finally spoke the truth out loud. The house was quiet, the kids asleep, and I sat on the edge of my bed, staring at the wall. My body felt numb, yet my heart pounded so loudly it felt as if it might burst.

In a trembling whisper, I admitted the words I

had been running from for so long: I can't do this anymore. This time, they felt very different. I had thought of these words often lately, but now, the words integrated, and I knew that they were very true and that, in my heart, it was over.

The moment those words were spoken, everything shifted. Suffocating fear took over because I knew admitting the truth would unravel the life I had been holding together by threads. At 43 years old, I was terrified to tell my parents and my family, AND they are my biggest cheerleaders, so I couldn't imagine sharing this news and announcing it to the rest of the world. It was absolutely terrifying.

And yet, beneath the fear, there was an unmistakable wave of relief. For the first time in years, I had spoken the truth to myself.

Then came the guilt. That crushing and relentless guilt.

What about the kids? What will people say? Am I selfish for wanting more?

Am I destroying my family?

I buried my face into my pillow and cried until there were no tears left, only the quiet rhythm of my own breath. In that stillness, I turned inward and spoke to the universe: *I can no longer do this. Guide me. Show me what I cannot yet see.*

And in that sacred silence, another voice emerged, softer, steadier than the guilt: You deserve to live fully. *You deserve to be seen. You deserve more than survival. You are the bridge of consciousness.*

In that moment, I realized something profound: the universe always meets us at the edge of our courage. Every fear, every moment of guilt, every trembling step forward isn't a barrier, it's a signal, a guide pointing toward where our next level of growth awaits.

I felt a wave of gratitude for the life I had lived, the lessons I had learned, the relationships that had both challenged and shaped me, and for the universe's gentle insistence that I was ready for more.

By honoring that moment, I began to reclaim my energy, my worth, and my power. Saying yes to myself didn't take from anyone, it elevated everything around me. The more I aligned with my truth, the more life reflected that alignment back: support, clarity, and opportunities appeared that mirrored the courage, value, and authenticity I was choosing to embody.

The breaking point became my breakthrough. What once felt like collapse became the foundation for expansion. And for that, I am deeply grateful, for the lessons, the relationships, and the universe showing me exactly where I needed to grow, guiding me into the life I was always meant to live. The patterns you resist most are the ones holding your greatest wisdom. Each one has served as a teacher, guiding you back to wholeness.

Leaving wasn't just for me. It was for them. Because children don't only inherit our DNA; they inherit our traumas, the way we live, the way we love, the way we either shrink or rise. Their dad and I had loved each other deeply once, and I don't regret that love. It shaped us, shaped them, and taught us lessons we carry forward. Sometimes, love takes a different form, evolving beyond what we first imagined. If I stayed small, unhappy, and invisible, I would be teaching them that this was normal, that this was love. But if I chose to leave, I could show them something greater: resilience, truth, courage. That night, I realized: Choosing myself was also choosing them.

What would shift if you chose to see leaving a relationship, friendship, situation, or job not as losing something but as expanding into something greater? Your children inherited not just your DNA, but your energy, your choices, your courage. What legacy are you leaving them?

The Motherhood Mirror

Motherhood has a way of magnifying guilt. Some days, survival was all I could manage, feeding them, driving them to school and activities, masking exhaustion with a smile when all I really wanted was to sleep for days. I compared myself to the mothers who seemed to do it all effortlessly: The ones with perfect hair and makeup at school pick-up, homemade baked goods in their children's lunches every day, homes that looked like they belonged in magazines. That pressure, and the guilt I carried for thinking I would somehow ruin my children's lives by choosing divorce, weighed heavily on me.

But one night after my separation, a moment changed everything. My oldest climbed into bed, studied me with those knowing eyes, and whispered, "Maman, you seem much happier now, and that makes me happy too."

Those words cut deeply. In that instant, the guilt, fear, and self-doubt evaporated. Children don't measure love by appearances. They feel energy. And he felt mine shift. He felt the truth. At that moment, I knew that everything would be okay because I was choosing it.

I realized then that leaving wasn't about abandoning them or regretting the marriage. It was about honoring the reality that we had simply grown apart. It was about showing them what it looks like to choose honesty over pretense, freedom over fear, and joy over obligation. In making that choice, I discovered not just my own liberation, but theirs as well.

I am profoundly grateful for my children, for every relationship that taught me something about love, and for the lessons that showed me exactly where I needed to grow. Each challenge became feedback, helping me strengthen awareness, boundaries, and self-trust.

When I started honoring my truth, I noticed real shifts, more energy, expansion and healthier relationships. Alignment stopped being a concept the moment I realized it lived in my everyday choices, in the words I spoke, the energy I allowed, and how I spent my time. Every yes and every no carried power. They weren't small decisions; they were energetic signals shaping my reality.

I began to pause before committing to anything and asked myself: Is this coming from alignment or from fear? Does this expand my energy or drain it? That simple check-in became a daily recalibration. It taught me to move with intention instead of impulse, to lead with energy instead of obligation. Authenticity turned into practice, not performance. It meant listening when my body asked for rest, honoring when something no longer felt right, and saying no without guilt. Those choices built strength from the inside out. My energy became clearer, and new opportunities started to align without force.

Choosing alignment over obligation is energetic leadership in action. It's how you show life the standard you now hold. Notice where your energy rises and where it drains. Protect what expands you. Set boundaries that reflect your worth. Every aligned choice upgrades your frequency, sharpens your clarity, and expands your freedom. This is how transformation begins, not by doing more, but by choosing from a higher state of being.

So I ask you: Which matters more, keeping up appearances, or living a truth that makes you feel alive?

What if survival isn't enough, and your soul is calling you toward the extraordinary?

Who might you become if you stopped apologizing for wanting more?

The Couch and the Calling

Around that same season, my then five-year-old had

a friend over. They ran through the house, wild and free, until they suddenly froze in the middle of our empty living room. The boy looked around, curious. "Why don't you have any furniture?" he asked.

I smiled. "We just haven't found the right one yet."

He paused, then asked with complete seriousness, "But... Do you have a toilet?"

I laughed. "Yes. We definitely have a toilet." That was enough. He shrugged, satisfied, and ran back to play.

To him, it was ordinary. To me, it was extraordinary. The old me would have spiraled: *What will people think? Am I failing as a mother? Am I falling behind? Will he tell his parents I can't even furnish a living room?* But instead, I felt a quiet, unshakable peace and true freedom.

Because I realized I was building something no one else could see. I was developing strength, resilience, courage, and trust. I was investing in my soul's evolution, not in appearances or things that didn't hold meaning. The furniture could wait. The image could wait. But alignment, healing, and truth could not.

In that stillness, I finally understood: what truly matters can't be measured by what others see. It can only be felt, lived, and chosen, now that is real freedom.

Here's what I learned: Life often gifts us moments that look like emptiness. Others may not understand what we're building, but the most important foundations are invisible at first. These are the foundations that hold everything else up when the visible pieces finally arrive.

If you're in a season when your "living room" looks bare, when others can't see the progress you're making, remember this: You're not behind. You're not failing. You're becoming. Every conscious choice you make, every boundary you honor, every act aligned with your truth sends a ripple of energy out into the world. That energy is what you attract back: opportunities, relationships, abundance, and growth that reflect the power you are cultivating within.

The universe always mirrors the energy you carry. When you choose alignment, integrity, and presence, you activate the power to quantum leap to transform your life in ways that visible accomplishments alone could never achieve. The invisible becomes unshakable, and, in time, the visible follows. Your choices are your power, your energy is your magnet, and your growth is inevitable when you honor the path your soul is asking you to walk.

True progress can be invisible at first. What matters most is the inner work, alignment, courage, and energy, not the immediate external results. How am I investing in the invisible foundations of my future success and freedom?

The Alchemy of Transformation

Abundance was never in what I could hold, it was in who I became while waiting, learning, and navigating detours that felt like delays but were divine direction. Every choice, every boundary honored or released, tuned my frequency, and the universe reflected it with perfect fidelity. True wealth lives in presence, in the energy you radiate, the shifts you spark, and the ripples you leave behind. Sacrifice is not loss, it's a sacred investment in becoming.

When I stopped chasing control and fully aligned with my power, I realized abundance is about the person I choose to become, moment by moment, and the frequency I embody. Fear never guided me; surrender, trust, and conscious choice did. Life reshaped itself not through force, but through alignment. Opportunities multiplied, energy expanded, my work soared, and my children witnessed resilience over fear. In that alignment, I became visible to myself, and that recognition was the true abundance I had been seeking.

Where are guilt, shame, or scarcity still holding you

back? Where are you performing for others while your soul quietly longs for freedom? What small or bold choice could finally shift your energy and your life?

You don't need perfect timing or permission. You need only the courage to listen, the willingness to choose, and the commitment to act, even imperfectly. Each conscious choice for yourself raises your energy, changes your reality, and models possibility for those around you.

Transformation is simple and profound: from guilt to confidence, from shame to self-respect, from survival to presence. The energy you carry shapes what you attract.

The universe mirrors your energy. Every choice today shapes the life you are meant to live. Every action aligned with your highest truth magnetizes growth, opportunity, joy, and quantum leaps. Your power to attract, elevate, and transform has always been within you, it's simply waiting for you to claim it boldly.

Reflection Exercises

Take a journal and spend some time with the following prompts:

- Where in your life are you still carrying guilt or shame that doesn't belong to you?

- If you peeled back that guilt, what would freedom look like?

- Where in your life are you still measuring your worth by what others see, rather than by who you are becoming?

- What's your "couch"? I.e., the safe, logical investment you think you need, but deep down, you know there's something bigger calling.

- How do you define true wealth, and how aligned is that definition with how you are living right now?

- What invisible foundation are you quietly building in your life that no one else may notice but that your soul knows is unshakable?

- How do I respond when life rearranges itself: with resistance or with surrender and curiosity?

Affirmations

I release the guilt that was never mine to carry. I choose worthiness in every breath. I choose visibility, even when it feels uncomfortable. I choose to be seen, known, and celebrated. I no longer hide from my own power and divine guidance, I embody it fully.

CHAPTER 4
IT ALWAYS BEGINS WITH YOU

"If you are always trying to be normal, you will never know how amazing you can be."
— Maya Angelou

Breaking the Rules I Was Told to Follow

I used to believe that if I just fixed the relationship, changed the job, or altered my circumstances, my life would finally fall into place. Yet every time, I found myself repeating the same patterns. External changes alone could never shift the energy. The real transformation began the moment I stopped looking outward and blaming others and started asking the harder, deeper questions: *What within me is asking to be healed? What is this person or situation revealing and reflecting back at me? What lesson is the universe delivering right now?*

This is radical responsibility. Not blame, not shame, not ego but power. Our emotions are powerful signals, showing us exactly where we are, where we are off course, and where growth is waiting. The instant you recognize that the shift begins with you is the instant you step out of victimhood and into authorship. You stop waiting for someone else to change, rescue, or validate you, and you remember that you have always been the answer. Life becomes a mirror, reflecting exactly what you need to see in order to grow, evolve, and reclaim your power.

There comes a moment when life calls for a radical choice: not to blame, not to dwell in shame, not to get lost in guilt or regret. Not because everything was your fault, not because you didn't try your hardest, and not because you didn't long for things to turn out differently. It might be the end of a relationship, the loss of a job, the collapse of a business, a health challenge, a friendship that fell apart, or a dream that didn't materialize. We often give everything we have, and sometimes, that simply isn't enough. And yet, "enough" is not measured by outcomes. It's measured by the courage to keep moving forward, to keep choosing, even when survival feels like all we can manage.

The journey is rarely simple. Some days are heavy, exhausting, and filled with doubt, grief, or fear. There are moments when you feel completely unsteady, unsure whether you can navigate life on your own or whether the decisions you're making are right. And yet, every emotion, every hesitation, every setback is feedback and an opportunity to pause, reflect, and course-correct. This is the power of conscious choice: it isn't about perfection, never making mistakes, or never feeling off-balance. It's about noticing, adjusting, and appreciating the guidance your own life offers, moment by moment, choice by choice.

So you choose differently. You stop outsourcing your power. You stop expecting someone else to fix your life or make you whole. You turn inward, to nurture yourself fully, imperfectly, and without conditions. You reclaim the parts of yourself buried under years of obligations, expectations, or self-sacrifice, whether as a parent, a partner, a professional, or a friend. You reconnect with your own curiosity, your own energy, your own voice. Before you can invite anything new, any opportunity, connection, or adventure, into your life, you must return fully to yourself: not the fixer, not the over-giver, not the one holding it all together, but the person you were always meant to be.

This choice is not easy, and it is rarely linear. But each time you make it, you step closer to living fully rather than surviving. Each time, you step closer to becoming the person your life is begging you to be and in doing so, you create space for the life, the love, and the opportunities you were always capable of receiving.

Each difficult moment, each uncomfortable emotion, each course correction became a catalyst for growth. By choosing alignment, integrity, and self-love, I shifted my energy, and the universe responded. Opportunities, abundance, and relationships that reflected my highest frequency flowed in. Every conscious choice I made multiplied my power, reshaped my reality, and created space for expansion. The energy you hold always attracts more of the same: growth, clarity, courage, and freedom. Your power is inherent, always present, and waiting for you to claim it. Choosing yourself, your truth, and your energy is the path to quantum leaps in life, love, and personal transformation.

I recognize that real transformation begins within me, not in changing others or circumstances. My emotions are my guidance system and show me where I am off course and where growth is waiting.

Dating myself for one full year

This wasn't a dare or a challenge I had signed up for online. This was about dismantling the walls I had built around myself for years and really turning inward, facing what I had avoided for years, peeling back the layers I used to hide behind, and learning to sit in my own company without distraction or escape. It was silence, discomfort, and real truth. It was the most rewarding thing I had ever done, but also one of the most difficult and uncomfortable. It was remembering the echoes of who I had been before I let myself disappear.

My family didn't entirely get it. Some of my friends didn't either. They tried, of course. They set me up, nudged me toward nice, eligible men. They looked at me with a mix of pity and puzzlement when I politely declined.

"Just go," they'd say. "You never know what might come of it."

But I did know. I wasn't ready, and I wasn't about to sit across from someone and pretend to be open when my heart was still healing. I didn't want to lead anyone on, least of all myself. The universe is not random: Every partner we attract is a mirror of where we are vibrationally. They show up to teach us, stretch us, and call us into the next best version of ourselves. That's why I made the decision to claim a frequency of power, self-trust, and unapologetic self-love. I wanted to stop attracting someone who needed me to fill their gaps, to soothe their wounds, or to complete their story, so that the universe would deliver a reflection of exactly that. Because when you align with your truth, the universe aligns the rest, and your relationships rise with you.

You are a magnet for the energy you carry. Before seeking connection, cultivate alignment, self-love, and inner clarity so that your relationships reflect the fullness of who you are, not what you feel you need to give or fix. Am I showing up in my relationships from a place of healing and power or from a place of seeking completion?

The Power of Solitude and Self-Recognition

So instead, I traveled. Alone, for the first time in years. I went to Haida Gwaii to see a close friend. On the way, I spent a few nights in Vancouver, one of my favorite cities. It was summer. The air carried salt from the Pacific, and the streets were alive with vendors, music, and laughter.

One night, I made a reservation at a restaurant by the water, a place known for its incredible sushi, the kind of spot you saved for a special occasion. I was totally worthy of it!

I walked in confidently: "Reservation under Angèle."

The hostess blinked, momentarily startled, then led

me to a window seat overlooking the harbor. The sky stretched wide in streaks of pink and gold, the water shimmering like liquid light in the last breath of day.

A few minutes later, the waitress arrived. She glanced at the empty chair across from me, then back at me with a kind smile. "Would you like to wait for your guest before ordering?"

I returned the smile. "Actually, I'll be dining solo tonight. Just me."

Her eyes softened, though I caught the flicker of confusion and maybe even pity. Not long after, another waiter stopped by. He looked at the untouched place setting across from me, then at me. "Are you still waiting for your guest?"

This time, my smile was steady. "Nope. Just me."

And I could feel his silent narrative: Poor woman, stood up, tragic, and eating sushi alone in a beautiful city like this.

For a moment, the old me wanted to rise up, to explain, to defend, to prove that I wasn't abandoned, broken, or invisible. To say: No, you don't understand. This isn't tragedy; it's liberation. I am not waiting for anyone. I am choosing myself and am finally free.

But I didn't.

I lifted my glass, focused on what was in front of me, and stayed grounded in my truth. Calm and freedom settled in me, clear and unwavering. Sitting there with my meal, I finally felt fully aligned with myself.

I wasn't lonely. I wasn't pitiful. I wasn't "less than." I was whole. I was enough. I was exactly where I was meant to be, and I will never forget that moment and that feeling of liberation!

That dinner was a statement of self-recognition. It reminded me that solitude is an opportunity to focus on my priorities, my growth, and the life I am creating.

I am whole, enough, and exactly where I am meant to be. By choosing myself first, I create a life that reflects my truth, my energy, and my highest potential.

Self-Love as a Magnet: Love Finds You When You Are Ready

As the year unfolded, that single night became a compass, guiding me inward. It led me to face the shadows I had avoided, the childhood wounds I had buried, the patterns I had repeated in love, and the fears I had projected onto others. The end of my marriage was no longer a mark of failure. It became a doorway, an invitation to rise, to reclaim the parts of myself I had abandoned, and to begin again with gratitude for the lessons, the relationships, and the growth that had shaped me into who I was and who I was becoming.

That evening taught me a truth I carry with me still: I am not waiting for someone else to complete or save me. I am enough. I am the company. I am the love I had been seeking all along.

Slowly, I felt ready to love again, not out of need, desperation, or a void, but from a place of wholeness, clarity, and alignment. I was open, grounded, and fully myself.

I began to imagine. I made a clear list and sent it to the universe, stating what I wanted: no young kids. My life is already full with three of my own. I'm driving to hockey and soccer games, packing lunches, juggling homework. I need simplicity. Ease. Someone older, someone emotionally and financially responsible. Someone adventurous, someone whose children are grown or who never had any. Someone who can meet me where I am, travel light, and love with freedom.

The universe delivered because our thoughts create our realities and what we focus on grows!

That summer, I met not one, but three men who checked every single box. All over fifty, all with grown adult children. Every detail aligned with what I had written and envisioned.

But here's the thing about specificity: It doesn't account for the unexpected, and it keeps the universe restricted to our requests when it can only deliver within that realm of our asking.

One invited me on a last-minute two-week adventure vacation. It was sweet, generous, the kind of spontaneous gesture that would have thrilled me. But I couldn't go. I had my children. I had responsibilities. My life didn't move on a whim.

So I let go. I released rigid lists, fixed expectations, and the illusion of control. I surrendered into trust, knowing that love would find me, not because I searched, but because I was ready. I rewrote my intentions for a partner, clear, expansive, and open, and trusted the universe to deliver in ways beyond my imagination.

The true transformation was never in the relationships I would form. It was in the love I cultivated for myself, the power I reclaimed, and the joy of fully inhabiting my own life. Sitting at a table for one, I recognized that I was already complete, whole, and worthy. That energy of self-respect, alignment, and trust became magnetic. It shaped my reality, attracted growth, and opened doors I could not have imagined.

This is the power of conscious choice: Every small decision, every moment of alignment, compounds into quantum leaps. It is not about perfection, but about consistently choosing yourself, your worth, and your truth. Your energy creates your reality. Every intentional yes to yourself amplifies abundance, clarity, freedom, and love, both for you and for those around you.

I am grateful for the lessons, for the reflections, for every relationship and challenge that showed me where I could grow. I thank the universe for guiding me toward alignment and readiness, for showing me that love, joy, and expansion are always available when we choose ourselves first.

Love finds you when you are ready. Not when you search. Not when you try to force it into your life. When you truly date yourself, when you honor your own worth, the universe mirrors that energy back, often in ways bigger, more beautiful, and more aligned than you could ever imagine.

Reflection Exercises

Take a journal and spend some time with the following prompts:

- When was the last time you did something just for yourself, without apology?

- When was the last time you felt completely at peace in your own company?

- What stories have you been telling yourself about being "alone"? How might you reframe solitude as spaciousness instead of emptiness?

- What patterns in love, family, or friendship do you notice repeating in your life?

- If your past relationship endings were not failures but invitations, what were they inviting you into?

- What rigid expectations might you need to loosen so that life (and love) can surprise you? Where in your life are you holding on too tightly?

Affirmations

I am enough, exactly as I am.
Solitude is not emptiness;
it is spaciousness for growth
and expansion.
I release the need to control
outcomes and allow the universe to
surprise me.

I am whole, and from this
wholeness, love will find me.
Every ending is an invitation to
return more fully to myself.

CHAPTER 5
RECLAIMING AUTHORSHIP
OF YOUR LIFE

---

*"When we are no longer able to
change a situation, we are challenged to
change ourselves." — Viktor E. Frankl*

Choosing Power Over Fear

For too long, I followed stories that weren't mine,
stories shaped by family, culture, fear, and outdated
expectations. They told me I was too much,
not enough, too ambitious, or too selfish. They
demanded that I perform to belong, shrink to be
loved, and settle to feel safe. The moment I took full
responsibility for my life, I realized that no one else is
in charge of my growth, my choices, or my outcomes.
That clarity shifted how I approach every decision,
every relationship, and every opportunity.

Living from your own values and intentions changes not only your path but also the environment around you. Each conscious choice reinforces your priorities, strengthens your focus, and builds a foundation for more honest interactions. Acting deliberately breaks old patterns and creates space for connection, trust, and consistent growth. Transformation is the result of repeated, intentional actions, not a single breakthrough.

Radical responsibility is not about being perfect or avoiding mistakes. It is about noticing your habits, evaluating your responses, and using life's feedback as information for adjustment. Every challenge, every uncomfortable feeling, and every difficult conversation is data that shows where growth is available. Each intentional action compounds, gradually increasing your influence, your clarity, and your ability to achieve outcomes aligned with your highest priorities.

Where are you still following expectations that don't belong to you? Which patterns are influencing your decisions without your conscious awareness? What one choice today can you make that prioritizes your values and strengthens your control over your life?

Growth is a series of deliberate choices. With awareness and accountability, you can break cycles, reinforce clarity, and expand what is possible in your relationships, work, and personal development. Your responsibility is the lever of change, and every moment is an opportunity to apply it.

I realized I have the ability to course-correct, to rise, and to claim my worth. For years, I lived on autopilot, reacting to circumstances, shrinking to fit expectations, or pushing myself to prove I was enough. I didn't fully understand that each choice I made, even the small, seemingly insignificant ones, shaped my growth and my reality. The moment I began noticing my patterns and acting intentionally, I saw the shift. Life started responding differently. Opportunities appeared. Relationships evolved. I felt the possibility of more, more growth, more abundance, more expansion because I was willing to take responsibility for my energy and my actions.

Mistakes have been a constant part of this journey. I've stumbled, misread situations, and sometimes chosen fear over alignment. What changed everything was learning to pause and reflect instead of judging myself. I asked over and over: what can I learn here? What does this moment teach me about my choices, my limits, or my desires? I began to celebrate the lesson in the mistake and the progress in the effort, rather than waiting for perfection. You can try this too: think of one recent challenge or misstep, how could you see it as an opportunity to act consciously and learn?

I've come to understand that growth is built through awareness, not perfection. Each time I notice a reaction, pause, and choose differently, I strengthen my confidence and expand my possibilities. I started asking myself simple questions: is this choice coming from fear or alignment? Am I acting to prove something or to honor my truth? Right now, identify one area of your life where you're reacting automatically. What would happen if you paused and responded with awareness instead?

Gratitude has been essential to this process. I've learned to recognize even small victories, acknowledge the lessons in struggle, and celebrate progress I might have ignored. By shifting my focus to what is working, what I'm learning, and what I'm proud of, I raise my energy and reinforce my growth. Take a moment now: what are three things you are grateful for today that reflect your growth, courage, or commitment to yourself?

Claiming my worth has been a practice I return to daily. I've had to learn to set boundaries, speak my truth, and act in ways that honor my values, even when it felt uncomfortable or met with resistance. Each time I do, I feel stronger, clearer, and more aligned with what I truly want. Reflect on your own life: where could you take one intentional step to claim your worth today, whether in your work, your relationships, or your personal life?

Every day, I remind myself that I am responsible for my growth. I have the ability to notice, adjust, and act consciously. Awareness is not always easy, and mistakes will continue to happen. But with reflection, gratitude, and intentional action, I create a life that matches the potential I know I carry. Begin now: what is one small action you can take today to respond consciously, elevate your energy, and move closer to the life you deserve?

When we elevate our frequency, we magnetize extraordinary outcomes, and align our life with the possibilities we were always meant to live. We can elevate our vibration, even when we are in the messiness of it, and make mistakes, as we celebrate the mistake and the growth through gratitude.

This is happening for my growth, and I have the power to respond consciously. I can notice, adjust, and learn. Growth is built through awareness, not perfection.

Radical Authorship

Before I stepped into my divorce, I made a vow that

this would not be destructive. This would not be bitterness, resentment, or lingering anger. I promised myself and my children that this ending would be a new beginning. It would be liberation. It would be a conscious choice. It would be a living lesson that endings are not failures, but gateways to growth, expansion, and freedom. I recognized the story society wanted me to carry, the shame, the sideways glances, the whispered condolences, the heavy sighs: "Oh, I'm so sorry, what a tragedy." As though divorce was a death sentence. As though my children were destined to grow up broken because their parents couldn't "make it work." That narrative was heavy, fear-based, and outdated. I refused to inherit it. I refused to let my children inherit it. I refused to make bitterness our legacy.

Radical authorship means taking full responsibility for your life and recognizing that you are the constant in every situation, choosing consciously in each moment, and aligning with your highest truth. It doesn't mean controlling others or owning their choices; you cannot dictate another person's actions, reactions, or behavior, only your own. Each individual carries responsibility for their own energy, decisions, and accountability. Your true power lies in how you respond, not in how others behave. Their choices do not define your worth or your alignment, only yours do.

When you step into this truth, the universe mirrors it back, amplifying your energy and opening doors to growth, freedom, and transformation far beyond what you can imagine.

But let's be clear, this isn't about perfection. We are human. We feel deeply. We get triggered. We fall into old patterns. We make mistakes. That's part of being alive. Radical authorship isn't about never faltering; it's about noticing when you do, meeting yourself with compassion, and choosing again. Every time you pause, reflect, and shift, you reclaim your power. You realign with your truth. You rewrite the story.

The goal isn't to avoid life's messiness, it's to honor it as the fuel for your evolution. Every stumble, every emotional wave, every uncomfortable moment is feedback, pointing directly to where growth is calling. When you meet these moments with gratitude, they transform into strength, wisdom, and resilience. True power isn't about getting it "right"; it's about staying awake to your choices, grateful for the lessons, and brave enough to choose alignment again and again.

Every yes, every no, every action taken in alignment with your truth compounds into profound transformation. The universe reflects the energy you radiate. When you fully embrace your power, trust your inner guidance, and act from alignment, abundance, opportunity, and expansion flow naturally into your life.

You are the constant in your own story. Your choices, not those of others, determine your power, your alignment, and your experience. Growth emerges through conscious response, never through control. Alignment is your practice, your strength, your superpower.

The Frequency of Choice

I refused to believe that the ending of a marriage meant I was broken. I refused to believe that my children's future was destined for tragedy. I chose instead to believe in endings with power, endings with grace, endings as intentional and beautiful as any beginning. Because life moves in cycles: it rises and falls, opens and closes.

It's not the ending that destroys us. It's the clinging, clinging to how things "should have been," clinging to the suffocating weight of other people's expectations, clinging to the story we once told ourselves. That is where disappointment festers. That is where our joy is stolen.

But when we let go and truly release with love rather than holding on with fear, endings transform. They become portals. They become gateways to new beginnings, to growth we never imagined. They do not break us. They awaken us. They launch us into exponential transformation.

So I set my intention: to lead with love. To lead with truth. To lead with integrity. To model for my children that relationships do not have to end in chaos, hate, or division. That even when love changes form, respect, kindness, and sacred bonds endure. That choice, aligned, conscious, fearless choice, is not failure. It's freedom, and the highest, most powerful expression of it.

This journey has not been easy. My ex experienced anger, and I understood why. Grief can show up as frustration, sarcasm, or resentment. I promised myself I would not respond with anger, hold onto bitterness, or allow negativity to influence my children. I am human, and I have made mistakes, but in every moment I failed, I asked myself why I was triggered and what I needed to address and heal. That willingness to face difficult emotions, learn from them, and act with intention and gratitude is where true growth lies. I am grateful for the lessons, for the clarity, and for the opportunity to become a stronger, wiser version of myself.

Your choices and your emotions directly shape your reality. When you meet mistakes with awareness, learn from experience, and acknowledge your progress, you elevate yourself and the impact you have on the world. Growth does not come from perfection. It comes from showing up consistently, examining your actions, and making deliberate decisions. Life calls you to take responsibility for your reactions and to make choices that align with your values and goals. Every conscious decision strengthens your ability to create the life you want and to move forward with clarity, confidence, and resilience.

Every moment is an opportunity to choose again. You are not defined by endings, mistakes, or emotions, but you are defined by how you respond to them. When you meet life with awareness, gratitude, and alignment, the universe mirrors that energy back, multiplying growth, love, and expansion in ways beyond what you can imagine.

Leading with Love, Grace, and Conscious Choice

I chose grace. I chose presence. I chose love and gratitude, even as everything around me was changing. In doing so, I showed my children that freedom is not a loss. It is a conscious choice. It is the ability to live in truth, to take responsibility for your well-being, and to lead with integrity.

What we model becomes the framework our children

live by. Words are temporary, but actions shape beliefs. I wanted my children to understand that you can disagree and still act with respect. You can choose a different path and still value the one that brought you here. You can close a chapter and still be thankful for everything it gave you.

This is the power of alignment and self-leadership. When we choose love over resentment, gratitude over blame, and awareness over reaction, we raise our energy and shift the world around us. The universe mirrors that vibration back through peace, opportunity, and deeper connection.

Life doesn't ask for perfection; it asks for presence and honesty. Growth happens when we notice, reflect, and choose again. Every moment is an opportunity to respond differently, to bring more compassion, more awareness, and more authenticity into how we live and love.

How can my actions, not just my words, reflect the values I want to pass on? In what ways can I respond with gratitude, awareness, and alignment even in challenging moments?

Redefining Endings, Reclaiming Power

When the news spread, the reactions were almost predictable (and, frankly, sometimes unbearable).

"Oh my God, I'm so sorry," they would murmur, eyes soft with pity, as if my life and my worth had just been condemned to some slow, tragic fate.

I would smile, sometimes laugh uncomfortably, and answer, gently yet firmly: "There's nothing to be sorry for. This is a good thing. This is best for all of us."

Some would blink, as if I'd just spoken another language. Others would sigh in relief, like a window had been flung open in a suffocatingly hot room. And I realized finally that their reactions weren't about me at all. They were mirrors reflecting their own fears, their own conditioning, their unspoken beliefs about what divorce means for them, through their lens.

Society and religion had led me to believe that the only "successful" family is the one that stays intact forever. Anything else? A failure. A tragedy. A loss. But I refused to live inside that myth and was certainly on a mission to spread a different truth.

At first, I kept my choice private, not out of shame, but out of awareness, caution, and strategy. I wasn't ready to carry the weight of everyone else's opinions. I knew most people meant well, but I also knew that even well-intentioned words can wound when you're still finding your footing. I would not let anyone talk me out of my truth.

I had chosen freedom. I had chosen presence. And nothing, neither their pity, their judgment, nor their fear could take that away from me. I refused to absorb other people's anxieties, and I refused to carry guilt for being responsible for my children's lives in a way that was aligned with my integrity. I was committed to my own alignment and to showing them through example that conscious, courageous choices are how we navigate life with strength, love, and clarity. And so until I had enough strength, I mostly kept it to family and close friends.

I needed space.

I needed clarity.

I needed to protect the sacredness of what I was choosing.

So I waited.

When I returned from a vacation, a colleague casually asked, "So, what did you do while you were away?"

I smiled. "I moved."

They blinked in surprise. "Oh? Where did you guys move to?"

I paused, steady, heart clear. "I moved out of our family home. We're getting a divorce."

The silence that followed was thick, almost heavy. They looked at me as if they weren't sure whether to hug me or offer condolences.

"Why didn't you say anything?" they asked.

And I told them the truth:

"Because I wasn't ready to hear what anyone else thought. I needed to arrive in my own clarity before I invited in the noise. Even if it went against the grain, even if it made others uncomfortable, I had to trust myself. This decision aligned with my heart and was not made from emotions, expectations, or paradigms."

And something unexpected happened.

People started opening up to me.

One by one. Quietly. Vulnerably. As if my decision had given them permission to say the things they had buried.

Some confessed that they were in marriages where love had long disappeared, but the thought of leaving felt too complicated and overwhelming.

Others admitted they stayed because of money, or fear, or judgment, and for the kids.

A few simply whispered, "I wish I were that brave."

I didn't feel brave. I felt human and vulnerable, and frankly terrified at times.

In that moment, I understood something profound: Courage is often just truth spoken out loud. And when I refused to shrink, when I chose love and my truth over the comfort of pleasing others or of looking good, I offered everyone around me a glimpse of a different possibility: a life lived fully, honestly, without compromise.

The truth is, we had tried. We had loved with everything we had. We had built something real. We had gone to couple's counseling. We had fought for us. But sometimes love doesn't end, it transforms. Sometimes it becomes friendship. Sometimes it becomes gratitude. Sometimes it simply becomes a chapter you carry forward, a lesson required for your evolution as you begin writing the next one.

And when your soul whispers that it's time to let go, not from anger, not from bitterness, but from truth and love, you have to listen and trust it because that voice will only get louder and louder until you finally face it. This is not just about marriage; this is about any life circumstance demanding your courage. Because life is now, is precious, and is far too short to spend being unloved, unhappy, or trapped in the shadows of what once was, or what others expect from you.

This was not my failure. This was not the end of my family. This was a different kind of ending, one that carried within it a beginning. A beginning of honesty, of freedom, of showing my kids and myself that sometimes the most courageous, the most loving, the most transformative act is to surrender what no longer serves.

And if I gave them nothing else, I gave them this: the proof that love can end without destruction, that endings can be graceful, that life can be lived fully even as one chapter closes. That lesson, the one I had learned through my own surrender, would ripple through their lives, touching every relationship, every choice, every moment they would ever face, long after mine.

Success is not measured by how long something lasts. It's measured by how consciously we move through it. Love that ends with honesty, grace, and gratitude is not a failure; it's a higher expression of truth. Endings can be sacred, relationships can evolve without destruction, and freedom can coexist with love.

Reflection Exercises

Take a journal and spend some time with the following prompts:

- Where in your life are you holding on because you're afraid of what others might think if you let go?

- How can I let go of what no longer serves me while honoring the past?

- In what ways has love in my life changed form rather than ended?

- What endings in my life have felt like beginnings once I looked back?

- What societal myths or pressures do I still carry, and how do they affect me?

Affirmations

I trust the wisdom of my own heart.

I give myself permission to create space, to breathe, to arrive at clarity.

I am not defined by endings, nor by what society expects of me.

I choose love, even when it looks different than before.

I am brave, not because I am unafraid, but because I speak my truth.

I allow relationships to evolve, to transform, and to teach me grace.

CLOSING OF SECTION ONE:

The Great Shift is about remembering who you truly are. Beneath the noise, the doubt, and the old stories, your strength, clarity, and power have always been present. By letting go of limiting beliefs, turning inward, releasing guilt, and embracing full responsibility for your life, you reclaim your authority and awaken to a fundamental truth: You are not broken. You were never lost, simply covered.

This is radical authorship. Every thought, every action, every choice is a vote for the life you want to live. Your energy, intentions, and actions are the common denominator in every relationship, every circumstance, and every outcome. The universe mirrors back the frequency you hold, rewarding alignment with opportunities, growth, and experiences that reflect your highest truth.

The Great Shift is not about perfection. It's not about never failing or never feeling fear, doubt, or grief. It's about noticing, acknowledging, and choosing again. Every challenge, every emotion, and every reflection is feedback, a chance to adjust, course correct, and grow stronger. Gratitude for these moments multiplies your energy and accelerates your expansion. Small, conscious choices compound into profound transformations over time, unlocking quantum leaps in personal, relational, and professional growth.

SECTION TWO
THE RETURN TO POWER

Enough of feeling drained. Enough of being stuck. Every challenge, every setback, every expectation is an opportunity to act consciously and reclaim your power. Life gives you moments to grow, expand, and step fully into your highest self. Mistakes and obstacles are not failures, they are stepping stones to the highest, best version of yourself. The more you recognize them, the more you transmute them into lessons, momentum, and quantum " leap transformation.

Your power is yours. It has always been within you. Stop giving it away. Own your decisions. Take responsibility for your energy, focus, and actions. Every challenge can be met with gratitude because it contains guidance. Every conscious choice compounds, elevates your life, and sets the stage for quantum leaping growth.

Surrender is not giving up. Surrender is alignment. It is acting with intention, courage, and focus. When you reclaim your energy, make decisions from integrity, and maintain clarity on your priorities, the universe responds. It mirrors your frequency with abundance, opportunities, and growth. This is the law: Your energy determines your results, and the universe matches your alignment.

Step forward with power, presence, confidence, and determination. Choose gratitude over frustration, awareness over distraction, and action over delay. Own your energy. Align your actions. Elevate your life. The universe is ready to match your frequency. The question is: Will you rise, embrace every lesson, and claim the extraordinary life you are meant to live and match it?

CHAPTER 6
BEGIN AGAIN:
THE ROAD MAP BACK HOME

"With the new day comes new strength and new thoughts." — *Eleanor Roosevelt*

I surrender into trusting that I am always taken care of.

I'll never forget one call, one that changed me forever. It came late, around 10 PM, the night before my new house was set to close. The final step. The edge of the finish line. I was exhausted, holding myself together with threads of hope and determination. For weeks, I had carried the weight of transition, the separation, and the uncertainty of new beginnings. And now, here I was, standing at the threshold of a fresh chapter.

My phone lit up on the nightstand. It was the

mortgage specialist, the woman whose voice had become a constant companion through this process. I had never met her in person, yet she had guided me through deadlines, signatures, and the chaos of logistics with patience and care. Her calm presence had been a lifeline when I felt fragile, a gentle reminder that support existed even in the storm.

I answered with a soft, "Hello."

Her voice carried a heaviness that made my chest tighten. "I'm so sorry to call this late," she said, pausing as though bracing to deliver a blow. "I have some not-so-great news."

My breath stopped for a moment.

She explained that, due to last-minute hurdles, lawyers, banking delays, and unresolved details from my separation, we were suddenly $2,000 short for closing. In the world of real estate, not a massive sum, but at that moment, it felt insurmountable. Without it, the closing might fail, and the seller's non-negotiable deadline loomed like a cliff.

As her words sank in, I looked around my childhood bedroom, the room I had retreated to when life had collapsed. I was back at my parents' home, after leaving behind the life I had built, the shared house, the memories, the belongings that once symbolized stability but now felt like chaos.

And then, in that stillness, a quiet shift occurred. I realized something vital: The universe always responds to the energy we emit. The fear in my chest? That would attract more scarcity. But the hope, the gratitude, the unwavering belief in the possibility of alignment, those energies would shape reality, too.

I took a deep breath and chose my vibration. I affirmed: *I am supported. What is mine will find me at the perfect time, in the perfect way.* I surrender and trust that all is happening for me always, even if I can't see it now and am devastated. I visualized the closing happening seamlessly, the money appearing exactly when needed, and felt a wave of calm certainty wash over me somehow.

I remembered one of life's greatest truths: We are what we attract, not what we want. If I carried panic and doubt, panic and doubt would meet me. If I carried trust, surrender, and resilience, the universe would mirror back those energies in miraculous ways.

I didn't know how it would happen. I didn't need to. I simply held the alignment, and I trusted the unseen. And as it turns out, the universe always responds to clarity, focus, and unwavering belief. That $2,000 appeared through an unexpected source.

Life often tests us in ways that feel urgent, critical, or even impossible, but these are the exact moments that reveal how we operate at our core.

Manifested Miracles

I had chosen to walk away, not because it was easy, but because staying would have cost me something far greater: my truth, my joy, my purpose.

That new house wasn't just a house. It was a miracle. The exact home I had visualized into existence, whispered about in quiet meditations, and written in journal entries during nights when trust was all I had. It felt like it had chosen me, like the universe had placed it on my path as proof that there was life after heartbreak, if you trusted in a higher calling and surrendered. And now, just hours before it was meant to be mine, it seemed like it was all coming to a dead end.

I broke down. The tears weren't only about $2,000. They were the weight of it all, the unraveling of a marriage, the painful logistics of separation, the endless decisions, feeling like a failure back at my parents' at age 43, the trying to stay strong when I felt anything but. This phone call felt like one more test, one more twist in the road before the new life could begin.

I sobbed into the silence.

And then, after what felt like forever, the woman on the phone spoke again. Her voice was softer now, almost angel-like, yet filled with conviction.

"I've watched you through this process," she said. "You've navigated it all with such grace, with fairness, with integrity, with love. I know it hasn't been easy. But you've done everything right."

There was a pause.

"I want to help you because you deserve it."

Confused, I sniffled. "What do you mean?"

"I'm going to lend you the $2,000," she said matter-of-factly. "You can pay me back whenever you can. I trust you."

I was stunned.

This woman, a total stranger, was offering me a miracle. Not because she had to. Not because she stood to gain. But because she saw me. Because she believed in me. Because, in that moment, she trusted me.

The tears returned, but they were different now. These were tears of gratitude, of awe, of disbelief at the kindness of the human spirit, the kindness of a total stranger I had never laid eyes on!

"I promise," I whispered through sobs, "I'll pay you back the moment the house closes." And I meant it with every fibre of my being.

That night, the weight lifted. What had felt like the end became another beginning. A miracle had arrived, delivered by someone I least expected, a testament to the universe's never ending support when you surrender to a higher force.

As I sat there in my childhood room, surrounded by the echoes of who I once was, a truth rose within me:

Life had not been working against me.

It had been conspiring in my favor all along.

Every heartbreak. Every closed door. Every detour that felt like failure had been leading me right here to this exact moment. To this reminder that trust, integrity, and love are the highest frequency, even when it feels like no one sees.

That night wasn't about $2,000.

It was about reclaiming authorship of my life.

It was about saying: I will not be defined by loss. I will not be reduced by circumstances. I will not let fear, scarcity, or doubt run my thoughts.

Instead, I will write my own story, one rooted in trust, love, and the belief that miracles are not accidents. They are responses to alignment and the frequencies we emit. This chapter of my life taught me that authorship isn't about controlling every detail. It's about choosing your response. It's about deciding who you will be when life tests you. Will you collapse into bitterness, or rise into faith? Will you outsource your worth, or claim it as your own?

When you choose love, gratitude, and trust, even when it's inconvenient, even when it's costly, the universe responds. Sometimes in quiet ways. Sometimes in breathtaking, miraculous ways.

That night, I didn't just close on a house.

I opened the door to a new beginning. Because that's what life is, one door always closing to allow another door to open. And when we resist the new door by holding on to the old, we block out amazing opportunities and magic that the universe is always pointing us towards and just waiting to gift us with.

True power is not control. It's alignment. Release the "how" and the "when." Trust that the universe will orchestrate the perfect outcome when you hold a high vibration.

Reflection Exercises

Take a journal and spend some time with the following prompts:

- How do you stay present when life's "miracles" are delayed or hidden behind obstacles?

- When you look back at a past hardship, can you see how it might have been guiding you toward growth or opportunity?

- How do you choose to interpret setbacks: as failure or as redirection?

- When have small acts of kindness or trust profoundly shifted your path?

- What frequency (thoughts, beliefs, actions) are you emitting that you want the universe to respond to?

Affirmations

I am the author of my life, and I
write it with love, trust, and courage.

Life is always working for me,
even when I cannot yet see the
bigger picture.

Every closed door is simply redirecting
me toward something greater.

I am worthy of miracles, grace,
and unexpected blessings.

I choose to trust the process
of becoming.

CHAPTER 7
SURRENDERING IS YOUR SUPERPOWER:
RELEASE CONTROL WITHOUT LOSING PERSONAL POWER

"When you let go of trying to control the outcome, you open yourself to miracles you never imagined possible." — Deepak Chopra

---

From Vision to Reality: Claiming My Life Through Bold Choices

I still feel the echo of my footsteps in that near-empty living room. Nearly a year had passed since I moved into my new house, and though it was bare, the space pulsed with possibility and held limitless potential, and I had consciously chosen that. The silence was not a void; it was an opportunity to expand into the next best version of myself. I recognized that this was a moment to make deliberate choices, to step fully into my vision, and to take ownership of the life I wanted to create. Everything I needed to build the life I imagined was available to me. I simply had to act with clarity, trust, and commitment, knowing that the universe supports those who move in alignment with their highest intentions.

I reminded myself that the power to shape my life is always in my hands. I can choose how I respond to challenges, how I prioritize my growth, and how I invest in my vision. Each choice I make from this place of trust strengthens my ability to create a life that reflects my true priorities, values, and purpose.

And so when I had chosen the leadership program over furniture, I had committed to moving forward fully. I had taken the steps required, made the investments needed, and trusted that the universe would meet me there, no doubt, and then some. I was no longer willing to wait for circumstances to feel convenient or for others to validate my choices or path. I had spent my life waiting for validation and arguing for my greatness in my marriage, so this was not about forcing outcomes or controlling every detail. It was about holding space for my exponential growth and alignment and knowing, in every fibre of my being, that everything I required would be provided at the right time.

The universe intervened in a way I could not ignore because I had asked intentionally, deliberately, in moments of quiet meditation what my next steps were, and the answer had arrived through a coaching program. Every dollar I had saved for furniture, every amount accounted went toward my expansion, growth, and transformation. The tuition had been high, a true stretch in every sense of the word, since it was in American dollars and my mind had screamed with fear at that time: "What will people think? Am I being selfish? Should I wait until life feels easier?" I had released old stories of sacrifice and "responsible" living and had placed my needs first this time because there was a fierce knowing that it was meant for me.

In that moment, I realized a profound quantum truth: Your life is the reflection of the choices you make from your highest vision, not your fears. The universe doesn't negotiate with hesitation. It responds to clarity, alignment, and bold intention. Every time you step into your vision, even when fear arises, you send a signal: I am ready. I am aligned. I am worthy.

I chose expansion over scarcity. I chose trust over doubt. I chose to invest in my growth, knowing that the universe is abundant, always providing exactly what is needed when you act in alignment. I reminded myself: Energy is magnetic. Vision combined with trust creates resonance. When you align with your highest self, the universe rearranges circumstances, opens doors, and delivers in ways the mind could never predict.

The empty living room transformed before me. It became a launchpad, a symbol, a tangible reminder that the life I imagine, the vision I hold, and the choices I make from alignment create my reality. Fear is a test, not a stop sign. Scarcity is a signal, not a sentence. And the universe is always, always ready to provide when we choose boldly, act from clarity, and trust beyond reason.

Choosing your vision is a declaration: I am ready. I am worthy. I am aligned. And in that declaration, every unseen support, every unseen provision, every miracle begins to move toward you. All that is required is the courage to choose your vision and then to step forward, fully aligned, fully trusting, fully ready to receive.

Because in this universe, what you choose in alignment, the universe delivers. Always.

Holding space for your growth while trusting the universe is the ultimate power move. You act intentionally while releasing the need to control every outcome.

Your Choices Shape Your Reality:
Fear Is Your Compass

The universe had opened a door, and my soul had been asked to step through. Trust. You are supported and loved beyond measure. Abundance flows to those who align with purpose, power, love, and, well, higher frequencies.

I had taken the leap at the time and had invested in myself. I had chosen growth over comfort, expansion over appearances. In that moment, I had declared to the universe that *I trusted the path forward and that what I needed would always come at the perfect time.*

Months later, there I was, unwrapping my living room furniture alongside my children, tears streaming down my face, not for the couches themselves, but for what that moment embodied. It was proof. Proof that transformation, surrender, and aligned action yield miracles. The leadership program hadn't just shifted me. It had cracked me open, ignited my purpose, sharpened my leadership, and deepened the bond with my children and my own inner power. And now, the universe delivered exactly what I was ready for, at precisely the right time. The furniture was more than furniture; it was a symbol of trust, alignment, and the magic of surrender.

I have learned to trust the timing of the universe.

What feels risky often arrives when you are ready for it. Scarcity is an illusion. Abundance is infinite, and it flows to those who lead with alignment, gratitude, and love. Follow your soul, not your ego, because what seems irrational is usually your next-level calling. Lean into your fear. It's your compass, pointing directly toward growth, expansion, and transformation. Practice radical gratitude, because every "empty living room" moment is a placeholder for blessings yet to come.

When you follow your intuition, even when it terrifies you, you unlock miracles, invite abundance, and align with the frequency of your highest self. The universe mirrors your energy. When you act from trust, love, and alignment, you magnetize exactly what you need, and often in ways beyond human imagination. Whether you realize it or not, your frequency is always attracting your reality. So why live in fear, scarcity, or frustration when you can radiate possibility, abundance, and expansion, and have the universe respond in kind?

Step boldly into the door before you. Empty living room? Tight bank account? The world telling you to wait? None of it matters. Align your heart, trust the process, and watch the universe deliver beyond your wildest dreams. Your next level is always on the other side of fear. Your miracles are waiting on the other side of trust. Say yes to growth, expansion, and your own magnificent potential. The universe is listening, and it always answers to the frequency you send.

Practice relentless gratitude for the journey. Every "empty living room" moment, every quiet pause, every leap into the unknown, is a placeholder for what is coming. Abundance is infinite. Trust is active. Growth is inevitable. Sometimes, all it takes is saying yes to the door in front of you, empty living room or not, and stepping fully into the extraordinary life that's waiting.

Reflection Exercises

Take a journal and spend some time with the following prompts:

- When has fear shown up as a guide rather than a barrier in your life?

- What opportunities are appearing now that you might be resisting due to doubt or social pressure?

- How can you practice trusting the unseen, knowing that the universe has your back?

- Where is scarcity speaking in your life right now? Write down three areas in which you feel fear, contraction, or "not enough." (Money, time, love, opportunities, etc.)

- Write down three times in your life when you took a leap of faith, even if it felt irrational, and were supported. Let those moments remind you that the universe has always had your back.

Affirmations

♡

I trust the universe to provide
everything I need.

I am always supported, guided, and
cared for.

I choose expansion over fear.

There is always more than enough.

CHAPTER 8
THE SACRED VOID: TRUSTING WHEN YOU CAN'T SEE

"Trust the wait. Embrace the uncertainty. Enjoy the beauty of becoming. When nothing is certain, anything is possible." — Mandy Hale

When Home Finds You: Trusting the Universe in the Unknown

Sometimes we don't find a home. The home finds us. And when it does, it feels less like moving in and more like a sacred remembering, knowing you were coming all along.

There comes a point in every journey when the only path forward is surrender. I found myself there, sitting in stillness, hands open, spirit weary yet hopeful and surrendering to a higher power. The weight of uncertainty pressed down on my chest at times, but beneath the heaviness, a quiet voice whispered: *Trust the universe. It always delivers more than you could possibly imagine.*

For weeks, I had been grasping for control, worrying about finances, logistics, and whether I would ever find a new space to call home for me and my kids. That night, I surrendered and told the universe that I was done and couldn't handle it anymore. I released everything since I was exhausted, tired and, frankly, totally depleted. *I'm ready for your support.* I didn't ask for just any house. I surrendered into *the house.*

In my mind's eye, a vision flickered. A giant window with radiant white light pouring in, a portal of peace and promise. A home close enough to my old neighbourhood that it felt familiar, yet far enough to mark a new beginning. It was never just about walls and floors. I longed for sanctuary. A place where my soul could exhale and expand.

At the time, logic told me this was impossible. During COVID, very few houses were available, especially in the neighbourhood I wanted, and the houses in my old adjacent neighbourhood were definitely out of my price range at that moment. Even the houses in the neighbouring community where I was looking to buy were priced hundreds of thousands of dollars beyond what I could afford. But if there's one thing I've learned, it's that the universe doesn't trade in logic. It trades in alignment.

Weeks later, I found myself with the real estate agent we had interviewed not that long ago when we were selling our family home. Though we hadn't chosen her then, something nudged me back to her now as though she was part of my story in a way I couldn't see yet at the time we first met.

We toured home after home. Each one lovely. Each one not mine. Each one way out of my price range.

Finally she paused, struck by a memory. "There's a house on this street that's not even on the market yet," she said. "An older couple owns it. The wife just moved into a retirement home, and the husband is overwhelmed with seventy years of belongings. I've been in touch with them for a while, but they have not listed it yet. Want to see it?" Without hesitation, I said yes.

The Frequency of Miracles

The moment I stepped into that house, my soul leapt in recognition. It wasn't polished. It definitely wasn't staged because it had mustard-yellow and green toilets, sinks, and bathtubs, all originals! But it was real. It had history and potential, and, most importantly, it had the light. That radiant, sacred light that had already appeared in my vision through the large, sun-filled front window in my meditation. I couldn't believe it at the moment but then paused and acknowledged my vision from earlier. I met the couple who lived there, and instantly, something deeper than chance bound us. The wife, frail yet graceful, spoke of her overwhelm, how impossible it felt to pack up a lifetime of memories with no support from her sons who lived far away.

An instinct rose within me. A knowing. I looked her in the eyes and said gently, "Why don't I buy the house, and you leave everything? I'll take care of it all."

Her eyes filled with tears. "I prayed for a miracle yesterday," she whispered, and here you are.

My throat tightened. My own tears spilled over. "I AM your miracle," I said, "because I prayed for one too."

In that moment, we were no longer buyers and sellers. We were two souls who had called each other forth through prayer in our collective field.

Logistics, of course, still loomed. The agent reminded me the house wasn't even listed yet, and my offer was far below the neighbourhood standard, nearly $300,000 less. But my soul knew and had nothing to lose at that point.

I made the offer.

And she accepted it on the spot!

Not because it made sense. Not because I forced it. But because I surrendered, and in that surrender, the universe moved on my behalf, carrying me exactly to what was mine. I declared, I visualized, I released my expectations, and I trusted in my heart that it was already done, that I was already taken care of.

Surrendering is not passive; it's active trust. It is choosing love, gratitude, and generosity over fear, doubt, or control. Life responds to the frequency you hold. When you align with your highest self and the universe, miracles arrive in ways that logic cannot predict, and abundance flows where it is most needed. Your life can always be elevated when you choose alignment, trust, and joy, every single time!

A House of Flow and Miracles

When I walked into my new home, keys in hand, it wasn't just my vision that greeted me. It was everything I needed and didn't have: kitchen supplies, furniture, plates, tools, water hoses, shovels, even art for the walls. Items I hadn't even thought to ask for, but which I deeply needed. It was as though the house itself had been preparing for me, holding space until I arrived.

The truth is that weeks before, when we had been

dividing items from our family home, I had been very generous in my offerings with my ex and unattached to material things, as I wanted to keep the peace and knew and trusted in my heart that everything would be delivered in divine timing when I come from love, gratitude, generosity, and joy. This is also a value that my parents instilled in me when our family home burned down when I was in high school. Material possessions are just material possessions, and what matters most is your health, your family, and your happiness.

To this day, I never get tired of sharing this story. My neighbour, a real estate agent, will sometimes still comment, "How on earth did you purchase your house in that price range again? That's unheard of!"

When you operate in higher frequencies of love, gratitude, and joy, abundance and miracles have no choice but to flow into your life and match your frequency.

Every moment is an opportunity to elevate your life by choosing alignment with higher powers and energies, over and over again. Surrender is not about giving up. It's about opening to limitless possibilities, trusting that the universe always has your highest good in mind.

This was more than a home. It was proof that when

you operate in higher frequencies of love, gratitude, and joy, abundance has no choice but to flow. When you choose alignment over control, when you declare your vision, trust in divine timing, and release attachment to the "how," miracles show up in forms beyond logic, beyond expectation, beyond what the mind can imagine.

I used to push through life as if effort alone could create what I lacked. I measured myself against invisible standards, forced outcomes, and ignored the signals that asked me to pause. I started asking: *Am I acting from fear or presence? What am I holding onto that no longer serves me?* That question changed how I made every decision.

Gratitude became a practice of noticing what already exists, the support in a conversation, clarity that comes from slowing down, ideas and resources I had overlooked. I began asking: *Does this choice expand me, or am I shrinking to feel safe?* Each answer guided my actions.

Intentionality required discipline. I started making choices based on what I truly needed, checking in with my body, listening to judgment, pausing before saying yes, and making rest a deliberate part of my routine.

Living this way changed everything. Joy appeared in

moments I hadn't planned, opportunities arrived I hadn't scheduled, and challenges became chances to reassess, notice resistance, and act consciously. Each day became a practice in awareness, gratitude, and deliberate choice. The more I acted intentionally, the more life responded in measurable and undeniable ways.

Reflection Exercises

Take a journal and spend some time with the following prompts:

- What "vision" or inner knowing have you had that seemed illogical or impossible yet continues to pull at your heart?

- Where in your life can you release control and make room for grace?

- Have you ever been part of someone else's miracle? What did it feel like?

- The Surrender Letter: Take out a journal/paper and write a letter to the universe. Begin with: *I release control and am open to receiving...* and list the things you're calling in: homes, relationships, health, opportunities. Be as vivid as possible and imagine how you will feel having it all. Then close your eyes, breathe deeply, and imagine placing the letter in the hands of something greater. Let it go and release your attachment, and so it is!

Affirmations

I surrender control and allow
miracles to meet me.

What is meant for me will
always find me.

I am ready to receive more than
I can imagine.

My life unfolds in alignment with
grace and in divine timing.

I trust the process, even when I
cannot see the outcome.

CHAPTER 9
THE TRUTHS OF ALL TRUTHS: SEEING BEYOND THE ILLUSION

"Between stimulus and response there is a space. In that space is our power to choose our response. In our response lies our growth and our freedom." — Viktor E. Frankl

The Power of Notice: Staying Grounded When Life Demands Everything

There are moments in life that imprint on your soul forever, moments that remind you how beauty and heartbreak can coexist all in the same breath. One of those moments came when I flew over 800 miles from home to be with my son while he received medical treatment in the United States. It was Mother's Day, a day meant for celebration, yet it carried the ache of separation. My heart was divided between being with my eldest and missing the laughter of my two younger ones who stayed behind. That weekend was both magical and heavy, a collision of gratitude and grief.

I woke up at the Ronald McDonald House surrounded by quiet compassion. Volunteers had prepared Mother's Day gift bags, each filled with generous treasures and immense care. I remember holding mine and crying, not for what it necessarily contained, but for what it represented: love, thoughtfulness, and the reminder that even in pain, we are held and thankfulness can exist.

Downstairs, by the coffee machine, I met another mother, a stranger who felt instantly familiar. She, too, was there for her child's treatment, her strength radiant despite the fact that she was missing a full limb. I wished her a happy Mother's Day, and without warning, tears filled my eyes. We spoke openly, two mothers baring our hearts, crying and smiling together in the raw truth of it all. In that sacred space, we became mirrors for one another, two souls recognizing themselves in shared vulnerability and power.

Later that day, when I returned from visiting my son at the hospital, a volunteer handed me a folded note. "We usually don't exchange contact information," she said softly, "but this woman insisted." Inside was a message from the mother I'd met that morning with her contact information. She wrote how our meeting had touched her deeply, and she offered something extraordinary: The next time I visited, she would pick up my two younger children herself so they could be close to me again. I sat in awe, tears streaming. The radical kindness of a stranger offering generosity even in some of her darkest moments, a stranger who was also driving with one fewer limb, and proof that when you don't let your circumstances define you, you are limitless and create ripples beyond what you could ever imagine.

One of my closest friends had flown in from Arizona just to be with me that weekend. His presence grounded me. He laughed, offered strength, and said, "Look at you holding space and creating generosity everywhere you go." In that moment, I felt it clearly: I was supported, not just by him, not just by strangers, but by forces larger than myself. I realized that when you truly surrender and let people support you, the support you receive goes beyond what you could imagine. It's a flow, a give-and-take, an abundance that moves in both directions. Even in receiving, we are giving. Something inside shifted that day. I saw a truer version of myself, stronger, more capable, and fully aligned with the support and abundance available when open to it.

Awake in the Storm: Awareness, Presence, and Inner Strength

Life was showing me that even in the middle of challenges and exhaustion, there are always miracles unfolding if we choose to see them. Gratitude invites them in. Presence expands them. Love multiplies them. And somewhere in that space between heartbreak and hope, I began to expand.

There comes a moment, somewhere beyond survival, when you begin to truly see yourself. It isn't detachment. It isn't numbness. It's awareness. It's the moment you recognize that you are not only the exhausted mother sitting beside a hospital bed, not only the woman filled with fear and praying for her child's health, but also the one who can see herself with compassion, clarity, and calm. You become aware of both the pain and the presence within you.

In the beginning, all I could do was react. I tried to fix everything, plans, schedules, outcomes. I carried everyone else's needs while ignoring my own. I braced for every beep, every shift in a doctor's tone, every new challenge, thinking that if I could control enough, I could prevent pain. But the truth hit me slowly, painfully: I could not control the situation, the doctors, the illness, or the world around me. The only thing I could ever control was myself: my response, my focus, my energy, and how I chose to feel in the midst of chaos.

I began to notice how my whole body lived in defense. Every time a monitor beeped, my stomach clenched. Every update from a doctor made my chest tighten. My mind stayed on high alert, scanning for what might go wrong, rehearsing every possible outcome. I was always preparing, always managing, as if control could protect us. Then one day, I caught myself. *This is fear*, I whispered. *This is my body trying to keep me safe.*

Naming it didn't change what was happening, but it gave me space for a breath between reaction and response. In that breath, I began to see the difference between control and love. I asked myself quietly, *What do I really need right now? Can I stay here, just in this moment, without running ahead to what I cannot know?* Sometimes I could. Other times, I couldn't. But even when the fear returned, it met a different kind of awareness. Something inside me had shifted.

That pause became a teacher. It showed me what surrender truly means, not the kind that gives up, but the kind that leads with trust. The kind that says, *I can't control this, but I can choose how I meet it.* From there, I began to trust that presence was its own form of power. I didn't need to plan every step to feel steady. I could breathe, listen, and stay close to what was real.

With surrender came quiet strength. I could sit beside my child without the storm inside me dictating every move. I could offer calm instead of worry, presence instead of panic. I learned that surrender isn't weakness; it's a return to love, to trust, to what matters most. Even now, when life feels uncertain, I return to that same question: *What can I release so I can meet this moment with love instead of control?*

And as I aligned with that choice, I began to notice something profound: the universe responds to alignment, not struggle. Support, guidance, and solutions arrived in ways I could never have manufactured myself. People stepped forward, doors opened, opportunities appeared, and I realized that when I release the need to control outcomes, I make room for the support, abundance, and clarity that are always available.

I learned a fundamental truth in those long nights by the hospital bed: The only thing I can ever control is myself, my energy, my focus, my decisions, my presence. Everything else flows in response to that. Fear, worry, and the need to fix are natural, but they do not dictate the outcome. What dictates the outcome is awareness, alignment, and the courage to respond deliberately, moment by moment. Surrender does not mean inaction. It means conscious action, fueled by clarity, trust, and the energy I choose to bring.

In learning to surrender, I discovered my power. I realized that even in exhaustion, even in the darkest moments, I am capable of steady presence, clear thought, and calm action. I am capable of receiving support and allowing others to give, creating a flow of abundance that strengthens both me and those around me. Every time I choose alignment over fear, awareness over reactivity, I claim my authority, expand my energy, and influence the world around me. Surrender became my strength, my strategy, and my doorway to living fully, even in the hardest circumstances.

I asked myself: Who am I beneath all of it? What happens when we step beyond our stories, beyond fear, doubt, and circumstance, and recognize that we are not defined by them but by the awareness we bring to each moment? That realization changes everything.

Growth begins when we stop reacting from fear and start responding from awareness. Life will always test us through loss, uncertainty, or change, but how we meet those moments defines who we become. When I chose compassion over judgment and acceptance over resistance, I discovered an inner steadiness that no circumstance could shake. That shift taught me that empowerment is not control; it's presence. Every moment, no matter how uncomfortable, carries a lesson and an opening to rise higher. The quality of my focus and the energy behind my choices shape my reality. When I approach life with gratitude, new possibilities start to appear. When I act with courage, things begin to fall into place. When I trust, expansion happens naturally. Each time I respond with intention instead of reaction, life meets me with clarity, opportunities, and a surprising sense of flow.

From Chaos to Clarity: Rising Into My Power

This is the power of awareness. The power of choice. The power to act with clarity, strength, and intention in every moment. By fully embracing this power, I step into a life of alignment, abundance, and limitless potential.

I learned the difference between experiencing an emotion and becoming it. Fear, anger, and doubt still show up, but they no longer run my decisions. They show me where I need to listen, change, or act. When I pause and ask, *What is this emotion asking of me? What truth is it pointing to?* I move from reaction to clarity.

Awareness is now my first response. I check in with myself: *What story am I believing right now? Is it real, or just familiar?* That question alone breaks old cycles. It reminds me I have a choice to respond from presence instead of habit.

From there, I focus on what I can control. I act on what matters, follow through, and make decisions that support the life I want. Each moment becomes an opportunity to practice discipline, courage, and direction.

What would change if you treated every emotion as information instead of identity?

What step can you take right now that aligns with who you're becoming?

Empowerment is built through consistency. It's choosing awareness over avoidance, progress over perfection, and accountability over blame. Alignment isn't something I wait for, it's how I deliberately create, decide, and choose to live every day.

Mindfulness, presence, awareness, they all lead to the same truth: healing begins when we observe without judgment. I learned that growth doesn't come from changing what happens, it comes from changing how

I meet it. I am not my fear, my doubt, or my pain. I reclaim myself by observing without judgment and choosing my response.

In that pause, I found my greatest power: choice. Challenge and presence can coexist. Fear and confidence can coexist. Grief and gratitude can coexist. Holding both brings clarity, focus, and control. And so ask yourself: *How am I showing up right now? What choice moves me forward?* Each pause is practice. Each decision shapes the life you intend.

Living at Full Potential: The Power of Focused Presence

Becoming an observer didn't just transform how I experienced specific challenges but how I experienced everything. I can face any situation with focus, intention, and alignment. I can act decisively, make empowered choices, and generate results that reflect my highest vision.

I am profoundly grateful for the pause that allowed clarity, for the perspective that revealed opportunity, and for the growth that strengthened me. I am grateful for the presence that softened me and for the capacity to hold space for my child, for myself, and for others. I recognize that expansion is not only personal; it is collective. When others hold space for growth, when communities support and align with one another, the energy multiplies. Abundance, clarity, and opportunity accelerate when we act in harmony, when we lift each other while we rise.

I've come to see that presence is where choice begins, and choice is where freedom lives. The way I show up in each moment, the attention I give, the decisions I make, shape not only my path but the person I am becoming. Challenges no longer feel like walls in my way; they are invitations to grow, to move faster, to become more of what I am capable of. Life responds to the energy I bring, to the focus I maintain, and to the alignment I cultivate. When I engage fully, clarity, opportunities, and growth show up naturally, almost as if they were waiting for me all along.

Choosing to stay present has changed everything. Gratitude grounds me, clarity guides me, and action carries me forward. In stepping fully into my awareness and responsibility, I realize the life I want isn't somewhere in the distance, it's something I create, moment by moment, in how I think, feel, and act. The more I engage with intention, the more expansive my world becomes, not just for me, but for everyone I touch along my path

Reflection Exercises

Take a journal and spend some time with the following prompts:

- Next time you feel triggered (fear, frustration, or control rising), pause for a single breath. Ask yourself: What am I noticing in my body right now? What am I noticing in my mind right now?

- Label the experience gently ("there's fear," "there's tightening," "there's a rushing thought"). End with the reminder: Between the trigger and the response, I always have a choice.

- Write down one moment when you were caught inside the storm (reactive, overwhelmed).

- Write down one moment when you were able to watch as the observer (aware, compassionate, steady). Reflect: What shifted when I was the observer? How did it change my experience?

- What am I grateful for in this experience? What did this experience grow in me (strength, patience, compassion, clarity)? Over time, notice how gratitude and growth can coexist with pain, expanding your capacity to hold both.

Affirmations

I am the observer of my inner world.

I can witness my emotions without being consumed by them.

I am whole, even in the midst of uncertainty and chaos.

I trust my presence to guide me through every storm.

I breathe, I pause, I reclaim my power.

I have the choice to begin again in every moment.

CHAPTER 10
LOVING OUT LOUD AND CHOOSING LOVE, ESPECIALLY WHEN IT'S HARD

"Your task is not to seek for love, but merely to seek and find all the barriers within yourself that you have built against it." — Rumi

From Pain to Power: The Mirrors That Launch Us

When my oldest was first hospitalized, I held on to hope, believing it would be temporary. I told myself we would be home soon. I thought this was just a short interruption, not a long-term situation. But days turned into weeks, weeks into months, and eventually, years. The life I knew changed completely, and I realized that control over the circumstances was not mine.

At first, that felt overwhelming. But then I recognized a deeper truth: The universe only gives us what we are ready to handle. Every challenge carries a lesson, a chance to expand, and an opportunity to grow stronger. What I could control was not the situation itself, but my response and how deeply and quickly I wanted to grow and expand.

It was in that awareness that everything began to shift. I started to notice mirrors all around me, reflections that revealed the parts of myself I had yet to heal. Being in the hospital, often alongside my ex, showed me where old wounds still lingered. Every silence, every tension, every awkward moment reflected my own patterns: the way I held my breath, softened my voice too quickly, or avoided conflict at all costs.

And then there was my son. He would get upset if I arrived even a few minutes late. At first, I dismissed it: five minutes seemed small to me. But to him, it was everything. Those minutes were a measure of love, presence, and attention. I realized that love is not about convenience but attunement. Showing up in the ways others need us, even when it's uncomfortable, is how trust and healing happen.

When I shifted my attention and chose responsibility over excuses, something remarkable occurred.

Healing began, not just for him, but for me as well. I started to see that every challenge, every tension, every reflection is an invitation from the universe: *grow, expand, step into the next best version of yourself.*

This is where most people miss how transformation happens, myself included. I had seen this over and over again and had coached hundreds of individuals, but this time I was seeing it through a very different lens as a loving mother watching her child endure such hardship. By noticing the mirrors, by observing the lessons, by responding with awareness, gratitude, and courage, we align with life itself. The universe responds. It matches our readiness with abundance, opportunities, and insight. Every challenge becomes a stepping stone, every lesson a launchpad.

I learned that growth is never linear. Pain is not punishment. It is preparation. When we meet life consciously, without blame, without avoidance, without resistance, we activate a quantum leap. Life no longer just happens to us; we begin to move in harmony with it, stepping fully into our power, our clarity, and our next level, and we begin choosing our experiences.

The hospital, the waiting, the tension, the guilt, they were all part of the process. They were not obstacles but mirrors, guides, and catalysts. And when we notice them, honor them, and act with presence, we are ready. Ready for expansion. Ready for abundance. Ready for everything the universe has been preparing for us all along, and then some.

Your Next Level Is Always Waiting for You to Notice

And here's one truth that will change everything: When you meet life fully, without excuses or avoidance, challenges become catalysts. Pain becomes power. Mirrors become guides. And you step into your next level, you quantum leap, ready to receive what the universe has been preparing for you all along.

That was the turning point: I stopped trying to fix everything. I stopped trying to control what I couldn't. My role wasn't to change what was happening; it was to love him through it. To hold space in unconditional, steady, non-performative love. To love him back to health. To love him back to life, as my closest soul friend would always tell me.

There was a woman, I think she was a teacher, who came to the hospital every day and read aloud to us for an hour. Just simple passages from books she loved and had chosen with my son's input based on his taste. Sometimes, I'd drift into sleep while she read, but her voice stayed with me, weaving a sense of normalcy into the cold hospital air. She may never know what a gift she gave us, but her quiet kindness reminded me of something essential: Sometimes, the smallest acts carry the most weight.

Her presence reminded me that healing isn't always loud or dramatic. Often, it's gentle. It's in the consistency, in the rhythms of presence, in the unspoken "I am here" without asking for anything in return. Healing also isn't linear. It comes in waves, forward and backward, messy and beautiful all at once.

After so much time in that hospital, I came to understand how easily we write stories in our minds of how things should be, of the lives we thought we'd have, but healing begins when we let go and accept the beauty of life as it is in that particular moment.

Love isn't always measured in grand gestures, but sometimes in presence.

It's the small gestures, the five-minute conversations, the shared silence. The reading voice in the room. The act of simply showing up. Time and presence are often the most profound expressions of care. Love is presence, not performance. It's not about fixing everything or having the right words. Sometimes, it's about sitting in the silence without trying to fill it.

Love doesn't always come with answers or fixes. Sometimes, it just asks us to stay. To hold space. To listen. To be there, on time, and with an open heart. When you lead with love, the universe has no choice but to match that frequency and return it back to you.

Reflection Exercises

Take a journal and spend some time with the following prompts:

- Where in your life are you trying to fix instead of simply love?

- How do you personally receive love? How do the people closest to you receive it, and are they the same?

- What stories about how life "should" be are you ready to release?

- Choose one person in your life today to show up for in a way that requires no fixing, no advice, and no performance. Just presence.

- Where in your life are you being invited to release control and simply be there?

Affirmations

I am enough when I simply show up.

My love is not measured in perfection, but in presence.

I choose to release the story of "should" and embrace the truth of "is."

I am learning to love myself as deeply as I love others. In every moment, love is available if I choose to be present.

CLOSING OF SECTION TWO

You are done waiting. You are done giving your energy away. Every challenge, setback, and moment of fear is an opportunity to act with clarity, take responsibility, and claim the power that has always been yours. Own your energy. Make deliberate choices from a place of focus, integrity, and alignment. Practice gratitude consistently. These actions create momentum, elevate your life, and attract opportunities, growth, and results.

Surrender is not giving up. Surrender is alignment. It is making decisions with intention, acting with courage, and maintaining clarity on your priorities. Every obstacle is information, every setback is guidance, and every challenge is a chance to improve. When you take responsibility for your energy, focus, and actions, the outcomes you seek follow naturally.

Step forward with confidence, presence, and determination. Choose awareness over distraction, action over delay, and responsibility over passivity. Own your energy. Align your actions. Elevate your life. The potential within you is unlimited. The extraordinary life you are capable of living is waiting. The question is: Will you rise and claim it?

SECTION THREE
THE RECLAMATION-ENERGY MASTERY

You wake up tired, already behind, running through the motions while life pulls you in every direction. Your calendar is full, the pressure never stops, and no matter how much you do, the clarity, energy, and fulfillment you want stay just out of reach.

I know that cycle. I lived it, driven by caffeine, deadlines, and the next accomplishment, yet still feeling restless, empty, and disconnected.Then it became clear: the problem wasn't my schedule. It was my **energy**.

Energy is the foundation of everything, how you think, how you lead, how you create results. When your energy is depleted, even small tasks feel heavy. When it's strong and aligned, everything becomes easier and more effective.

The moment I took full responsibility for my physical, emotional, mental, and spiritual energy and stopped giving it away to obligations, overcommitment, and constant striving, everything changed. Mistakes became data. Challenges became momentum. Progress accelerated

When you manage your energy first, you perform better, think clearer, and move through life with power and purpose. You stop reacting and start leading. You stop surviving and start expanding to let in what truly matters.It all begins with one decision: to take back control of your energy.

This is The Reclamation.

It's the conscious shift from surviving to thriving. When you align with your highest self, clarity, abundance, and freedom are inevitable. Opportunities show up. The right people enter your life. Your resilience grows. Your life expands beyond what you thought possible.

As you rise in alignment, you create space for what truly matters, more joy, more peace, more purpose. You begin to do less, yet achieve more. By clearing what no longer serves you, you open your life for expansion and invite the new to enter. You become more efficient, more powerful, more magnetic than you've ever known. What once required force now flows with ease, and you complete things in a fraction of the time, because you're no longer pushing against life, you're aligned with it.

If you are ready to step fully into your power, your focus, and your highest alignment, your time is now. Take ownership of your energy. Commit to your growth. Elevate your life. Rise. Align. Transform. Your quantum leap starts the moment you decide.

CHAPTER 11
THE RECLAMATION:
MANAGING YOUR ENERGY,
NOT YOUR CIRCUMSTANCES

"Energy cannot be created or destroyed. It can only be changed from one form to another."
— *Albert Einstein*

Intentional Presence: How Challenges Propel Transformation

The first time I stepped into the ICU as a mother, I felt the huge weight of responsibility, but I also felt clarity, purpose, and power. Every monitor, every machine, every alarm reminded me that my focus and presence mattered. Every breath my child took demanded conscious attention, and in that demand, I realized a truth: I always have a choice. I can respond with fear, or I can respond with intention, determination, and action. In choosing presence, I step into my power and can be exactly where I need to be.

At the same time, life continued at home. My two energetic boys moved through their days full of life and wonder, and I felt immense gratitude for the unwavering support of my parents, my sisters, my friends, and my community. They helped with meals, school runs, errands, sports activities, and every detail that allowed me to focus, to act, and to grow. Their love and presence reminded me that I am never alone, that every moment of support fuels my ability to rise higher.

The hospital has its own structure, and within that structure, I found focus, discipline, and resilience. Morning rounds, medications, tests, and alarms demanded my attention and required me to show up fully. Nights were long, and in that time, I strengthened my endurance, remembered my vision, and trusted that I was growing into the next best version of myself moment to moment. Every challenge became a measure of my capacity. Every obstacle required deliberate action and commitment to growth.

This is alignment in practice. Every day, every moment, I have a choice. I can react with fear, frustration, or exhaustion, or I can respond with clarity, presence, and purpose. When I respond from a place of emotional intensity, when I falter, I can choose again. Every second is an opportunity to adjust, refocus, and take control of my energy, my intentions, and my actions. Life does not require perfection. It requires awareness, deliberate decision-making, and the ability to course correct, moment by moment.

There were days when everything felt overwhelming, when every new task or decision felt like proof I wasn't enough. I used to react quickly, emotionally, sometimes out of fear, and it always left me exhausted. Slowly, I began to notice something different. When I paused, when I showed up fully present and acted deliberately, things changed. Opportunities appeared that I hadn't seen before. Insights came when I took the time to notice them. I realized alignment isn't a one-time achievement. It's practice. It's making choices with intention, taking responsibility for my energy, my focus, my reactions, even when everything is hard. The more I stayed present, the more clarity and results I saw. Looking back, the difference was in the small, consistent choices, the pauses, the reflections, the deliberate actions. They didn't just change outcomes; they changed me forever and what I attracted back into my field .

The Paradox of Hospital Life

Hospital life is a paradox. You feel trapped, yet expansive. Exhausted, yet more awake and present than ever. Grieving, yet filled with gratitude. Terrified, yet discovering a strength you never knew existed. And yet... not everything inside that life is dark.

You find intentional ways to create joy: watching movies, piecing puzzles, drawing on gloves with Sharpies, laughing at the absurd moments only hospital life can bring.

You create rituals, you build connections, you make meaning, and you shape a home away from home, and resilience is born, the kind that grows day by day, in those unseen moments. The kind that proves your spirit cannot be confined, even by four hospital walls, the strongest of them all.

People often say, "I don't know how you do it." The truth is, neither did I. And yet, you do. Because love, especially the love for your child, makes you capable of the impossible. Timelines lose meaning. Fear transforms into focus. You stop clinging to what you cannot control and start investing fully in today. Every small victory becomes monumental. Every moment becomes sacred. Hope anchors you, and gratitude fuels you.

Surrender is strength. Letting go of control is not weakness. It's a superpower. When you release, you make room for grace, clarity, and unexpected opportunities. Presence outweighs perfection. A held hand, a kind word, a quiet moment, a hot cup of tea— these simple acts shift everything. Connection heals and reminds you that love is always present, even in the hardest moments when you choose to notice them. Gratitude transforms. Seeing compassion, support, and love in chaos reshapes your energy, expands your heart, and amplifies your power.

Challenges aren't roadblocks, they're catalysts. Every difficulty reshapes you, stretches your capacity to love, and expands your power to rise beyond limits. Each moment of fear, fatigue, or doubt is quietly preparing you for your next evolution. You survive, and in surviving, you ascend. You rise stronger, wiser, more grounded in truth and aligned with purpose and power.

You are not behind. You are exactly where you're meant to be. Every challenge is momentum. Every breath is mastery. Every act of love is a signal to the universe that you are ready for more. This is the paradox and the gift of life: even in the hardest moments, you are expanding, ascending, and becoming unstoppable and limitless.

Beyond the Box: Rising Through Life's Challenges

In moments when the weight feels unbearable, it is natural to focus solely on survival. But those moments are also the ones that shape your capacity for resilience, clarity, and intentional action. Choosing presence, focus, and gratitude allows you to transform every challenge into a catalyst for growth.

Here's the truth most people miss: The universe doesn't give you challenges to make you suffer. It gives you challenges to wake you up. Every time you say, "I can't handle this," you are right because the version of yourself you've been until now may not be capable. But the higher version of you, the one life is calling you to become, absolutely can. The universe is not asking you to carry the weight as the person you have been; it's asking you to rise into the person you are becoming. That shift begins the moment you stop asking, "Why me?" and start asking, "What is this here to teach me?"

Growth is not automatic. Many people live the same year repeatedly and call it a life. Pain alone does not transform you; your willingness to learn from it does. You always have two choices: resist, fight the lesson, numb the pain, and stay stuck in survival mode; or allow, open to the lesson, let it stretch your faith, and grow into a version of yourself you could not access otherwise. When you choose growth, challenges become accelerators, and pain becomes power. What you once feared or resisted becomes the key to your evolution.

No matter the challenge, whether illness, loss, divorce, or uncertainty, you have the power to choose your perspective and your response. Survival is not the goal. You are not here to simply get through life. You are here to accelerate and quantum leap. Every challenge is an opportunity to grow stronger, wiser, and more capable. In the ICU, watching my child fight for life, I learned that strength is not about never struggling but choosing presence, focus, and intention. At the same time, life continued at home with my two energetic boys. Their busy routines and ways of lighting up a crowd reminded me that life moves forward, and the unwavering support of my parents, sisters, friends, and community allowed me to act with clarity, prioritize what mattered most, and engage fully.

You are capable of handling more than you realize. Every challenge, setback, and moment of pressure is an opportunity to rise, to grow, and to expand your capacity. You always have a choice: Resist and stay stuck or engage fully, learn the lesson, and step into a stronger, wiser version of yourself. Resistance becomes resilience. Setbacks become setups. Pain becomes power. Pause and ask yourself: "What energy do I choose in this moment?" Reframe your challenge: "What is this teaching me?" Anchor in your future self, stronger, clearer, freer, and let that perspective guide your decisions today.

When you engage fully, choose growth, and practice gratitude, you move beyond survival into acceleration. You step into the person you were always capable of becoming, stronger, clearer, and fully aligned with the life, love, and purpose that are ready for you now. The universe is not here to break you. It is here to reveal your potential. Your hardest moments are accelerators, shaping clarity, strength, and purpose.

Reflection Exercises

Take a journal and spend some time with the following prompts:

- When life feels like it has placed me "in a box," how can I choose presence over perfection in this moment?

- What small rituals, connections, or moments of gratitude can I create to anchor myself in resilience today?

- Where in my life am I still trying to control what is uncontrollable, and what would surrender make possible?

- How has adversity expanded me, deepening my empathy, patience, or capacity to love?

- If I stopped asking *how long* and started asking *what matters right now,* how would that shift my perspective?

Affirmations

Even inside the smallest of boxes, my spirit expands. I choose surrender, presence, gratitude, and growth. Love makes me capable of the impossible.

CHAPTER 12
MAGNETIC WEALTH

---

*"Abundance is not something we acquire.
It is something we tune into." — Wayne Dyer*

From Trigger to Treasure

I'll never forget the day I was tested in public view for everyone at work to see. It was an ordinary hospital day with a very full waiting room in our department, and eyes were gazing all around. I was walking out of my office when a man stormed towards me. He didn't soften his tone. He didn't hesitate. He looked at me with a sharp stare and said words that cut through my gut:

"You are the reason your child is in the hospital. It's because of you. Because of your choices. Because of your divorce."

I couldn't breathe. My whole body burned with

shame, anger, and disbelief. I stood frozen, trying to comprehend what was happening. He had actually come to my workplace, to my place of safety and purpose to tell me that it was all my fault. All of it. The words hit like a slap. The urge to defend myself rose fast and hot, a tidal wave of anger and pain. *How dare you?* My mind raced with arguments, explanations, the desperate need to correct his story and reclaim my dignity.

But in that suspended moment, something shifted. Beneath the noise of my thoughts, a quiet awareness surfaced. I saw that his words were not really about me. They were the reflection of his own turmoil, his pain, his fear, his need to project what he could not hold within himself. His frequency was fear, and fear always seeks somewhere to land, someone to blame. If I reacted, I would only join him in that frequency, matching his chaos with my own, and handing over the power that was mine to keep.

So I didn't. I took a breath that steadied me from the inside out. I felt the tremor of restraint, the strength in my stillness. Then I smiled, calmly and deliberately I asked him to leave. Softly, but firmly. I chose peace over ego.

That moment taught me something unforgettable: the situations that challenge us most are invitations to rise above reaction. They show us exactly where our energy wavers and where growth is asking to happen. When you learn to recognize those moments, they become powerful mirrors guiding you back to your own frequency, to freedom, to power.

Love, Gratitude, and Joy as the True Path to Abundance

Every trigger is a teacher. Every mirror reflects exactly where you stand, where old pain still lingers, where strength has already taken root, and where your power is being refined. The universe doesn't send judgments to punish you; it sends reflections to awaken you deeper. Each challenge is a frequency check, a spotlight on the next layer of growth waiting to unfold, if you choose it.

Triggers don't just expose the wounds; they reveal the healing. They illuminate how far you've come, how deeply you've expanded, how resilient you've become. Every flash of discomfort is an invitation to rise higher, to embody your evolution, to meet yourself at a new level of truth and grace.

That was me the day he stormed out of my workplace. I didn't defend, explain, or shrink. I simply stood still anchored in gratitude. Not gratitude for him, but for myself. For the power I had cultivated.

For the growth I had earned. For the quiet knowing that required no proof, no defense, only presence, true FREEDOM at last.

Every thought, word, and action you put into the world carries a vibration. That vibration shapes the quality of your experiences and the opportunities that appear or disappear around you. You are not a victim of energy; you are its source. You generate it with every choice you make.

Your frequency can be adjusted at any moment. Awareness is your power. When you practice intentionality, you shift from living on autopilot to living on purpose. You begin to notice the thoughts you entertain, the language you use, the activities you choose to engage in, and the energy behind your actions. Each moment becomes a chance to realign, to raise your frequency and move closer to the life you want to create.

Gratitude is one of the highest frequencies you can live from. It's not just a feeling; it's a state of energetic alignment. It's one of the most powerful ways to shift your energy. Gratitude is not just an emotion; it's an energetic accelerator. It rewires your focus from what's missing to what's working. It trains your mind to see opportunity where others see limitation. It magnetizes more of what resonates with joy, peace, and expansion.

Intentionality and gratitude are simple daily practices. They require awareness, repetition, and choice because simple does not always mean easy. But the more you align your energy with clarity, purpose, and appreciation, the more magnetic you become. Life begins to respond differently. Opportunities unfold. Support appears. You feel grounded, empowered, and connected to something greater than circumstance.

Remember that your energy sets the tone. When you choose to live intentionally, to speak consciously, to act with awareness and to lead with gratitude, you become the frequency of what you want to attract. And life can't help but meet you there.

Vibration Over Circumstance

It hasn't always been this way for me. You're not "in control" of your emotions or not, like flipping a switch. Growth isn't linear; it rises and it falls and sometimes it tests you. That's where accountability, perception, and responsibility become your superpower, your chance to course correct and try again.

I got here because I chose to quiet my mind. Year after year, I invested in intuition, in connection, in the universal god source that lives inside me, and inside of you too. When you pause long enough through meditation, presence, and mindfulness, your vibration rises. Your higher self speaks, you can hear it, and clarity flows. Answers don't come from the outside but emerge from the divine universe you carry inside. True knowledge and wisdom can't be handed to you. They are cultivated and embodied.

Every challenge, every interaction, every mirror you face is here to elevate you, to expand you, to push you into the next best version of yourself. When you see it this way, energy rises. Quantum leaps happen. You see what you're attracting and that you have the ultimate control over what you are calling into your experience, gaining the power to shift it and course correct it if needed.

Even when you're triggered. Even when you stumble and fall flat on your face with everyone watching. Even when you respond in ways you later regret, this is true freedom, and gratitude transforms it. Every misstep shows you where to grow. Every reset is a gift, and cultivating gratitude even in these moments elevates your frequency.

The way forward isn't about fighting the old. It's about embracing the new. Every new moment is a choice: align with the solution or feed the problem.

Elevate your vibration and attract abundance by

intentionally recognizing and amplifying what you appreciate. Gratitude is a vibration multiplier. The more you notice and cherish, the more the universe mirrors it back in abundance.

The Frequency of Abundance

The universe will always respond to your energy. It will always mirror back the frequency you hold. And when you choose love, gratitude, and joy, again and again, the universe cannot resist. It rises to meet you with opportunities, with relationships, with miracles, and yes, even with the money that supports the life you're here to live. I have come to recognize that when you surrender and ask the universe for catalyst shifts and growth, it provides exactly what you require for your spiritual expansion.

I understood loud and clear that life responds to our energy, our frequency, and matches what we put out in the field. We have a choice in every single moment in how we'll choose to respond, no matter the trigger or how big. We choose how we'll respond, where we place our focus, and what energy we carry into the world, and it returns to us. In every moment, you have the power to create something new, a new moment, a new opportunity.

Energy is contagious. Choose carefully what you expose yourself to. Choose high-frequency environments and people that amplify your growth and abundance.

Your Frequency Creates Your Reality

Love transcends all, and every time you choose love over hate, especially when it's hard, life opens wider and paths appear along the way to assist you. Gratitude multiplies, what you cherish grows, and the more you notice, the more the universe pours out in return. Fear contracts, pulling life inward, narrowing vision until opportunities right before your eyes vanish into shadows. The universe always matches your frequency. At the foundation of all creation is vibration. Everything you experience, every thought, every emotion, every interaction, is an energetic exchange. Your emotions are not random; they are your most reliable guidance system. They mirror your vibration and reveal whether you are in harmony with who you truly are or resisting that alignment.

Align your inner frequency with the life you want to attract. The universe responds to the vibration you hold internally before anything material appears externally.

Energy Is Everything

Every thought carries energy. Every word you speak and every emotion you hold sends a signal that shapes your reality. Life reflects what you project, nothing more, nothing less. If you want abundance, clarity, and peace, you must deliberately choose higher states of energy: love, gratitude, and joy, again and again.

Love keeps you centered when ego wants control. Gratitude cuts through negativity and shifts your focus to what's real. Joy elevates your energy so you can create, lead, and move forward. The real test isn't when life runs smoothly, it's when judgment hits, when things fall apart, when fear takes the wheel. Those moments define your frequency. Choosing love when it's hardest, gratitude when it feels undeserved, and joy when nothing justifies it, that's where transformation happens.

Over time, these consistent choices build an unshakable foundation. They condition your body, heart, and mind to return to love automatically. Eventually, it's no longer a conscious practice, it becomes who you are. That's the frequency of real freedom. That's where abundance stops being something you pursue and starts being your natural state.

"Your energy introduces you before you even speak."
— Anonymous

Small, consistent practices compound. Your life transforms when alignment becomes habitual, not occasional. Daily practices of reflection, gratitude, and energy alignment create unshakable abundance.

Reflection Exercises

Take a journal and spend some time with the following prompts:

- What moment today tested my energy? How did I respond?

- Where could I have chosen love, gratitude, or joy over fear or judgment?

- How did small, high-frequency choices today create positive shifts in my experience?

- What patterns do I see in the energy I attract and project? Rate your energy from 1–10 and note any patterns: what elevates you and what drains you?

- How can I strengthen my ability to respond consciously instead of reacting? Anchor words: Pick one word for the day (e.g., LOVE, GRATITUDE, JOY, POWER) and return to it whenever your energy dips.

Affirmations

Abundance surrounds me in every form: love, money, opportunity, and growth. I am the master of my energy; I choose what I create.

Every thought, word, and emotion I emit aligns me with my highest self. My vibration shapes my reality, and I consciously cultivate it with love, gratitude, and joy. Each moment is an opportunity to elevate, reset, and align with my highest path.

CHAPTER 13
YOUR ENERGY IS YOUR HIGHEST CURRENCY: OWN YOUR ENERGY AND CREATE ABUNDANCE

"What you think, you become. What you feel, you attract. What you imagine, you create."
— Buddha

From Control to Clarity

I used to think success meant control, control over my schedule, my outcomes, even my emotions. I believed that if I worked hard enough, stayed disciplined enough, and managed everything perfectly, life would eventually reward me with peace, satisfaction, and fulfillment. But the harder I tried to control, the more I lost myself. I was exhausted, performing constantly, chasing a balance that never arrived.

Then life hit me with challenges I could not plan for, push through, or fix with sheer willpower. Everything I relied on achievement, productivity, structure, suddenly failed me. In that moment, I realized something life-changing: fulfillment does not come from controlling circumstances. It comes from mastering your energy, how you think, how you feel, and how you respond to what life brings.

You cannot control everything no matter how hard you try, but you can control your inner state, your thoughts, your energy. You can cultivate awareness, consciously choose your responses, and elevate your frequency. That is where clarity, resilience, and power are born. Life will always bring the unexpected, but when your energy is aligned, you no longer just survive the chaos, you thrive in it.

This awareness marked the beginning of a profound shift. Instead of asking, "How do I fix this?" I began asking, "How do I want to feel, and what would support that feeling?" That single question became the foundation for a new way of living, one based on the frequency of my energy, awareness, and choice.

This chapter explores the concept of Energy Mastery, a practical and conscious approach to living that goes beyond time management, productivity, or external success. It's about understanding how your energy shapes your reality, how your emotions serve as your internal guidance system, and how caring about how you feel can become the most powerful way to quantum leap success in your life and attract quantum growth.

The Foundation of Fulfillment

Ever wonder why some people seem to have it all and thrive in every area of their lives, health, relationships, career, and overall joy and fulfillment. It can be tempting to assume they work harder, have better luck, or simply have more time. But the truth is that their success is not determined by time, luck, circumstances or effort alone. The key difference lies in how they manage their energy. Time is limited, but energy can be renewed, expanded, and directed with intention.

Through my own journey, I've learned that fulfillment does not come from managing time or controlling every detail. It comes from managing energy, being intentional with thoughts, emotions, and actions. The way we use our energy directly shapes the quality of our experiences. Every interaction, decision, and mindset choice affects how we feel and how effectively we move through life.

We live in a culture that rewards performance,

productivity, and perfectionism. Success is often equated with endurance, control, and the ability to stay strong no matter what. Emotional awareness, vulnerability, and self-compassion are too often viewed as weaknesses rather than strengths. This belief system leads many people to disconnect from themselves, ignoring the signals their emotions provide. In reality, our emotions are essential indicators of where our energy is flowing and whether we are aligned with what truly matters.

For years, I believed success depended on time management and effort. I convinced myself that working harder, doing more, and maintaining control would lead to happiness and fulfillment. My worth became tied to my productivity and the ability to meet external expectations. I filled my calendar with commitments and goals, yet internally I felt drained and disconnected. I was functioning efficiently but living without alignment. My focus was on managing time instead of managing the energy behind my actions.

The power of committed action became one of the greatest catalysts for my transformation. As a natural doer, consistency and discipline were already familiar to me, so I decided to channel that focus into my inner work. For seven months straight, every single morning, I sat in our basement to meditate.

For seven months, I practiced stillness. I tried to quiet my mind, to connect to something greater, and to remember who I truly was. At first, it was extremely difficult. I felt that meditation was not my gift and that I was not a natural at it. I wanted to give up. My mind raced constantly with tasks, plans, and endless thoughts. I felt restless, uncomfortable, and frustrated that I could not slow down.

Despite the difficulty, I continued to show up every morning without fail. I committed to the practice even when it felt impossible.Then one morning, something shifted. The noise in my mind stopped. I felt a calm I had never experienced before. In that stillness, I heard a clear, quiet message from within: **Your energy determines your reality**.

The message struck me deeply. I did not fully understand it at the time, but I recognized its importance and truth. From that moment on, I began to take responsibility for my energy. I aligned my choices with my state of being and started to lead from a place of awareness and presence.

That moment changed everything. It became the foundation of how I live, lead, and create. I learned the value of showing up consistently, with discipline and trust, even before clarity arrives. To this day, I remain profoundly grateful for that guidance and for the realization that taking responsibility for my energy shapes every aspect of my life.

After that turning point, I began paying attention to where my energy was going. I noticed that every thought, task, and relationship either supported or depleted me. Certain patterns, overcommitment, people-pleasing, perfectionism, and constant digital stimulation, consistently left me feeling exhausted. On the other hand, activities such as meditation, movement, presence, time in nature, and genuine human connection consistently renewed me. Once I recognized this pattern, I began to make conscious adjustments.

To build awareness, I started tracking my energy each day like a bank account. I identified which experiences filled up my energetic bank account and which one depleted it. Seeing the results in writing brought clarity. I realized that I often gave away my energy unconsciously, saying yes when I meant no, holding on to guilt, or ignoring my emotional needs. Taking responsibility for protecting my energy was not selfish. It was necessary. Over time, my relationships deepened, my productivity improved, and my energetic reserve expanded. You can complete work tasks and everyday demands in a fraction of the time when you operate from that space!

Energy management is not about perfection or maintaining constant positivity. It is about self-awareness, recognizing when your energy dips and taking small, deliberate steps to restore balance. Emotions play an essential role in this process. They provide information about whether you are aligned with your values and truth. When you learn to listen to your emotions instead of resisting or suppressing them, you can realign your energy quickly and effectively.

Life will always bring challenges, uncertainty, and change. Resisting these experiences only creates more strain. Growth begins when you accept what is happening, learn from it, and adjust your energy and mindset accordingly. The ability to pause, reflect, and choose a different response is a sign of power and self-mastery, and every single person has access to that too, including you! When you make choices from awareness instead of fear or reactivity, you reclaim control over your energy and the direction of your life.

Your energy is your responsibility. No one else can protect or manage it for you. The more intentional you become about how you think, feel, and act, the more aligned your life becomes. The people, opportunities, and circumstances around you begin to reflect the energy you cultivate within yourself.

Energy management is not just a personal tool but a life philosophy. It shapes how you lead, connect, and create abundance everywhere.

When you make caring about how you feel a daily priority, you strengthen your emotional intelligence and create the conditions for quantum leaps in growth and transformation. You become more present, grounded, and balanced, able to respond to life with clarity instead of reacting out of habit or stress. This is what true empowerment looks like. It is not about doing more; it is about accomplishing more with a fraction of the effort. It is about aligning your thoughts, emotions, and actions so they work together in harmony, amplifying your results and your sense of purpose.

Energy and Empowered Living

I had worked intentionally for years to manage my energy and had coached hundreds of people on how to master theirs. My life felt balanced, aligned, and abundant. I was creating my reality with clarity and intention. But as life often reminds us, growth rarely happens in comfort. When my eldest child faced serious health challenges, I was thrown into a new level of testing and transformation. Months and months in and out of hospitals forced me to become even more intentional with my energy, to learn how to manage it differently when everything around me felt totally out of my control and chaotic.

At first, I felt isolated, as though I was the only person navigating that level of pain and challenge. But over time, I realized that while no one had my exact experience, everyone faces moments that challenge their strength, perspective, and ability to stay grounded. The greatest lesson I learned was that no one else is responsible for my peace, happiness, or energy. No circumstance, person, or outcome, no matter how challenging, can determine how I feel unless I allow it. When I believed life was happening to me, I gave my power away. When I took ownership of my energy, no matter what was happening around me, I experienced freedom, clarity, and a strength that came from within, even in my darkest moments. That was when I truly understood surrender and that we create our realities, even in chaos and when life brings you to your knees, especially then. The universe is always looking out for us through experiences.

Life will always unfold in unpredictable ways. Change, challenges, and uncertainty are inevitable parts of being human. Resisting them does not stop them; it only amplifies frustration and drains your energy. Transformation begins when we stop resisting and start embracing what life brings. Every experience, even the painful ones, expands our capacity and raises our energetic vibration. When we meet life with openness instead of fear, the universe mirrors that openness back to us through growth, alignment, and opportunities we could never have imagined ourselves.

Mastering My Energy, the True Measure of Success

We live in a culture that measures success by output, how much we do, how fast we move, how much we achieve. But constant striving often disconnects us from our own energy and truth. Real success is not about doing more and controlling more; it is about being more aligned. It's about cultivating awareness of how our energy feels and learning to realign when it shifts out of balance.

We are not meant to maintain high energy all the time. Life flows in natural rhythms. There will be peaks and valleys, expansion and contraction. What matters most is the ability to recognize when we have slipped into lower frequencies like fear, anxiety, or control, and to consciously return to balance. Growth is not about avoiding difficulty. It's about shortening the distance between reaction and mindful response.

Every moment gives us the opportunity to begin again. To pause, breathe, and realign with who we truly are. That mindfulness of our thoughts, emotions, and energy is what transforms everything. Spending so much time in the hospital supported me in finding deeper truth to energy mastery as I had to learn to master mine so that I could be there for my kid.

I started being very intentional with managing all my bodies as best I could so that I could be there for my child in hospital, but also there for my other younger two boys at home. I took care of my physical body through enough sleep (and yes, often that was a nap in the hospital bed or chair or a movie cuddle with my younger two), rest, movement, and nourishment. I strengthened my energy foundation and also worked on nurturing my emotional body by noticing whether my feelings stemmed from gratitude, love, control or fear, and I realigned as required.

I worked on my mental body by focusing on what I wanted to grow, change and spend my energy on with mindset shifts (e-books, podcasts, mindfulness, etc.). And I surrendered to spirit, to God, to source in a radical way by constantly asking to be shown the way with purpose, integrity, and alignment with my higher self, so that my life could flow with more ease amidst the chaos.

Energy is influenced by everything we interact with in our environments: relationships, conversations, and even the content we consume. The more intentional we are about these choices, the stronger and more stable our energy becomes. Every challenge I have faced has reminded me that I alone am responsible for my energy. When I chose awareness over reaction, growth over resistance, and presence over perfection, I reclaimed my power.

I spent countless hours in the hospital by my eldest's bedside, watching monitors, waiting for updates, and holding my breath with every change in his condition. At first, I tried to control everything. I tracked every chart, asked every question, and focused on tasks, believing that if I stayed busy, I could keep us safe. I pushed down my emotions, thinking that appearing strong was necessary. Over time, I realized that I could not control the outcome, and resisting that truth only exhausted me. The only thing I could control was my own energy, how I chose to respond, how present I could be, and how I could care for myself even in the midst of uncertainty.

As I focused on my energy, I noticed the difference it made. When I consciously chose awareness, gratitude, and calm, I was more effective, more patient, and more connected to my child and the people around us. Even small moments, a smile, a kind word from a nurse, a quiet pause, felt significant. I began to understand that challenges were not simply obstacles, but opportunities to practice presence, responsibility, and intentional action. I learned that even when emotions ran high or circumstances felt out of control, I still had the ability to choose how I responded.

Through this process, I realized that the energy I carried shaped my experience. When I prioritized rest, mindfulness, gratitude, and boundaries, I was able to respond more clearly and intentionally. Support and kindness appeared in response to the energy I held, and I saw that my own consistency and clarity had an impact on the people around me. My child's journey became a teacher. I became a more capable mother, a more resilient person, and a clearer presence in every relationship.

I now understand that energy matters more than anything else. It is not about controlling outcomes, but about managing how I respond, how I stay present, and how I care for myself. Spending so much time in the hospital taught me that even when I cannot control circumstances, I can control myself, my attention, and my choices. That control became the foundation for my strength, my clarity, and my ability to navigate life with intention and focus.

Energy in Motion: Finding Balance Through Chaos

The happiest and most successful people on the

planet are those who master their energy. They are intentional with their thoughts, emotions, and habits. They choose their company wisely and cultivate gratitude consistently. The universe speaks in energy: It communicates through synchronicities and signs that mirror what you are ready to receive. When your frequency is grounded in appreciation, kindness, and love, you naturally manifest what supports your highest good.

Gratitude became my anchor throughout my son's health journey. It didn't change the situation, but it changed how I experienced it. It helped me see the blessings that coexisted with the pain and the strength that emerged through the struggle. Gratitude transforms perspective; it shifts energy instantly and magnetizes solutions, support, and peace.

Energy mastery is a daily practice. It requires awareness, choice, and courage. You are 100% responsible for your energy and, therefore, for the reality you create. Every "yes" or "no" you give is an energetic statement that shapes your life. Saying yes when you mean no creates energetic leaks that drain your vitality. Setting boundaries preserves your energy and communicates to the universe that you are operating from self-respect and alignment.

Your outer reality reflects your inner state. Taking control of your energy is not optional. It is essential. Every thought, feeling, and choice shapes the results you experience. When your energy is focused, clear, and intentional, everything in your life aligns accordingly.

Protect your energy. Notice what drains you. Eliminate what doesn't serve you. Double down on what strengthens and inspires you. Set boundaries, prioritize your focus, and make choices that keep your energy high. Every action matters because energy drives results.

Your energy is your most valuable asset. Guard it, cultivate it, and use it deliberately. When you master it, you master your life. The clarity, focus, and results you want are no longer a matter of chance but are a direct reflection of the energy you choose to bring, no matter what life throws your way.

Returning to Alignment

Energy Mastery is not a destination; it is a daily practice. Every moment offers a choice to react unconsciously or to respond with awareness. When you begin to observe how your energy moves, you realize that your emotional state is not random; it is information. It tells you where your attention is, whether your thoughts are aligned with your truth, and if your actions reflect your values.

Caring about how you feel is not indulgent. It's what separates extraordinary living from reactiveness. It allows you to pause before exhaustion sets in, to recalibrate when your energy feels scattered, and to reconnect with what matters most. The more you prioritize your internal state, the more stable and grounded your external world becomes.

Energy Mastery begins with awareness, expands through consistency, and becomes effortless through alignment. The more you honor your emotions, protect your peace, and make choices that reflect your highest values, the more you begin to experience extraordinary living, not as a concept, but as a lived reality.

Your frequency is the foundation upon which everything in your life is built. When you learn to manage it with intention, you don't just improve your circumstances. You quantum leap change and transform into extraordinary living in every area of your life.

Reflection Exercises

Take a journal and spend some time with the following prompts:

- Where in your life could you take ownership instead of waiting for circumstances to change?

- What fears are showing up when you consider stepping into your next level?

- How could slowing down and listening to your intuition accelerate your growth?

- Who or what has shown up in your life as a reflection of the energy you are putting out?

- Where in your life do you feel your energy being drained?

- How can you choose one action today that supports how you want to feel? What activities, environments, or relationships restore you?

Affirmations

I am in full control of my energy, my attention, and my choices.

My thoughts, emotions, and actions are aligned with my highest good.I cultivate gratitude daily, and it transforms my perspective and my life.

I honor my boundaries, protecting my energy and my peace.

I respond to life with awareness, clarity, and intention, not reaction. My energy shapes my reality, and I choose it consciously and courageously.I release what drains me and focus on what strengthens and inspires me.

CHAPTER 14
RADICAL RESPONSIBILITY: MISTAKES ARE NOT MISTAKES. THEY ARE GROWTH PLATFORMS TO ABUNDANCE

"You attract what you are, not what you want. If you want great things, then you must become a great person." — Abraham Hicks

---

People don't break you. They reveal you

I've learned one simple truth: How you show up changes everything, how you live, how you love, and how you grow. For years, I thought setting intentions, praying, journaling, and repeating affirmations would be enough. They weren't. Real change comes from noticing your energy and how it shapes your choices, your words, and your actions, in combination with your intentions.

When I got married, I wanted a loving partnership, but I hadn't healed the parts of myself that doubted my worth. My energy carried both hope and fear, and life reflected both back. Over time, I learned to take responsibility for my energy, believe in myself, and align my actions with what I wanted to create. Life shifted. Opportunities, relationships, and experiences arrived that supported my growth.

Your energy matters. When you nurture it, life responds. You have the power to create your reality and show up fully, for yourself and for those you love.

Every person who enters your life, every triggering moment, every sharp word or unexpected judgment are all mirrors. Sacred, sometimes painful, mirrors showing where your inner work remains to be done. And yet, these mirrors are also portals to your greatest growth. They are the universe's way of guiding you toward your next evolution.

Here's the mindset shift: You are exactly where you are meant to be in your soul's evolution. Every challenge, every person, every circumstance is aligning perfectly with your growth, even when it doesn't feel comfortable. When you welcome these experiences and ask the universe for guidance, clarity, and signs, you activate the highest law of creation: You call in exactly the people, situations, and opportunities your soul needs to expand.

You create your reality through the energy you carry. You do not attract what you think you want; you attract the vibration you embody. When you heal, align, and raise your energy, life reflects your highest self. The universe never makes mistakes. It responds to the frequency you hold. Every person, every situation, every challenge is exactly what your soul needs to grow. Pay attention. Ask for guidance. Notice the signs. Be conscious of your choices and the energy you project.

You are not broken. You are becoming. Every challenge, every interaction, every reflection shows you how far you have come and directs you to where you are meant to go next. Your energy determines your experiences. When you stay aware, intentional, and aligned, you attract what truly matches your highest self. There is no delay. There is no mistake. You are exactly where you are meant to be, and every moment is an opportunity to evolve, rise, and call in what serves your growth.

Accountability as Freedom

During my son's hospital stays, I was stretched to my limits, juggling shared custody, hospital visits, and caring for our two younger boys. Life demanded everything from me. Then one day, his father told me he believed it was my fault he hadn't received the promotion he wanted. He said the time spent navigating our divorce and family challenges had made him less present at work, less able to travel, and that the opportunity had slipped away.

At first, I was stunned, angry, even. How could I possibly be responsible for someone else's career or choices? But instead of reacting, I took a breath, paused and listened. I held space for his frustration without taking it on as my truth.

And in that moment, something powerful shifted. I saw my evolution reflected back to me. I realized I no longer needed to defend, justify, or absorb someone else's projections, especially his. I understood deeply that each of us is the creator of our own reality. Our energy, choices, and focus shape our results.

That moment wasn't about blame, it was a mirror showing me my own growth. By responding with awareness, compassion, and clarity, I embodied my truth: I am responsible for my energy, my path, my peace, my freedom. It was a defining moment of power and liberation, proof that when you stand rooted in accountability and self-awareness, you no longer bend under the weight of someone else's story. You rise above it, anchored in your truth, freedom and expansion.

This experience reinforced a powerful truth: We create our reality through our choices, energy, and awareness. The people and situations we encounter are opportunities to measure our growth and exercise conscious decision-making. When we take full responsibility for ourselves, stay aligned with our values, and act intentionally, we attract experiences that reflect our highest self. Every challenge, every interaction, and every moment is a chance to choose consciously and shape the life we are committed to living.

I understood that your power isn't in controlling others. It's in choosing your frequency, especially when it's hardest.

My son's health challenges and time in the hospital were among the most difficult moments of my life. Yet, in the midst of fear, uncertainty, and exhaustion, I discovered a profound truth: even in the most intense circumstances, I could master my energy. Every moment tested me. Every interaction and every challenge presented a choice, fear or trust, resentment or gratitude, blame or responsibility. I chose presence and gratitude.

I began noticing joy in the smallest moments, a

kind word from a nurse, a shared laugh, a quiet breath of relief. I felt the support of those around me and witnessed acts of generosity that reminded me that love and connection are always available, even in difficulty. Time spent with my ex became a space for healing and clarity, a space where growth was possible for both of us and for our son. Every situation became an opportunity to deepen awareness, strengthen presence, and align with a higher frequency of energy.

This journey revealed a powerful reality over and over again: **your energy is your most important resource**. Every thought, word, and reaction either fuels your growth or drains your vitality. When you hold onto resentment, your energy diminishes. When you blame, it dissipates further. When you act from love, your energy rises. When you speak and stand in truth, your energy compounds. The universe responds not to your circumstances but to the energy you carry.

I've witnessed this countless times working with patients facing serious illness. Two people can face the same diagnosis and the same circumstances, yet their outcomes are entirely different. The difference is not the situation, it is the energy they choose in response.

Ask yourself: **What am I choosing today?** Fear or trust? Blame or responsibility? Automatic reaction or conscious response?

The truth is, your energy matters most when it is hardest to choose. Life is smooth sometimes; it is easy to stay positive when everything is going well. The real test, and the real power, emerges in moments of challenge. In those moments, the energy you cultivate shapes your experience, your growth, and the impact you have on everyone around you.

Take full control of your energy, protect it deliberately, and raise it consistently so that you do more than survive challenges; transform every difficulty into a source of strength, clarity, and progress in every area of your life. Examine honestly where you are holding yourself back, recognize where growth is required, and understand that personal development is a process that requires persistence, reflection, and intentional action, not a straight path. Every challenge is an opportunity to take responsibility, make conscious choices, and align your thoughts, emotions, and actions with the person you are committed to becoming. You are not a victim of circumstances; you are a conscious creator and fully responsible for shaping your reality, and the power to act, rise, and thrive exists in these very moments.

Reflection Exercises

Take a journal and spend some time with the following prompts:

- When I feel triggered or judged, what part of me is actually being revealed?

- Where am I still giving away my energy: through fear, blame, or old stories?

- How can I shift from reacting to consciously choosing my frequency in this moment?

- What "deposits" into my energy bank would strengthen me today? (Gratitude, truth, compassion, boundaries.)

- If I fully believed I was a deliberate creator, what would I stop tolerating or carrying that drains me?

Affirmations

I am the creator of my reality, and I choose my frequency with intention.

Every trigger is an invitation to heal, grow, and return to love.

My energy is my currency, and I invest it only in what expands me.

I release blame and reclaim my power. I am responsible for my healing and my abundance.

The universe always rises to meet the vibration I hold, and I choose alignment, clarity, and love.

CHAPTER 15
SIGNS, SYNCHRONICITIES, AND SOVEREIGNTY: THE UNIVERSE IS ALWAYS RESPONDING

"Synchronicity is an ever-present reality for those who have eyes to see." — *Carl Jung*

Fear as a Path to Freedom

There are moments in life when clarity doesn't come from planning, logic, or careful strategy, but from stillness, surrender, and the courage to trust yourself. I have learned that these moments are rarely comfortable, rarely predictable, and often require that we step into fear. One such moment came to me during meditation. I was shown two large key holders, each brimming with keys, different shapes, sizes, and colors. Some were ornate, some simple; some shiny and new, others worn and familiar. I stood there, hesitant, noticing myself overthinking every choice. Which key would open the "right" door? Which choice would lead to the "perfect" outcome? Fear whispered that I needed certainty, control, and a guarantee that nothing would go wrong. And then it became clear: There is never a wrong key. Every choice, even the uncertain or risky ones, carries lessons, growth, and opportunity. Every decision moves you forward, even when you cannot yet see where it will take you.

Leaving my marriage was one of the most difficult and terrifying decisions of my life. I had no idea what the future would hold. Uncertainty stretched in every direction: the logistics of co-parenting, the emotional upheaval of separation, the financial pressures of managing a household on my own, and the deep fear of stepping into a life I had not yet built. Every day was filled with questions that circled endlessly in my mind: Was I making the right choice? Could I handle the responsibilities that were about to shift entirely onto my shoulders? Was I risking too much, and what would the consequences be for me and my children?

Despite all the fear and doubt, I recognized that staying would mean sacrificing my sense of self, my growth, and the life I wanted to create. I committed to a year of focused healing and self-discovery, intentionally exploring who I was beyond the roles I had carried for so long, mother, wife, employee, and reconnecting with my own values, desires, and voice. Each step forward, no matter how small, felt terrifying in the moment, yet every choice I made to prioritize myself, my healing, and my growth became a catalyst for transformation that I could not have anticipated.

I learned to navigate fear not as a signal to retreat, but as a guide pointing toward the areas where I needed to grow, stretch, and expand. The process was not linear, and there were days of doubt, exhaustion, and grief, but each of these moments taught me resilience, self-trust, and the power of deliberate action. I discovered that the decisions that feel most impossible, the leaps that provoke the deepest anxiety, are often exactly the ones that propel us toward our greatest growth.

Trust, Action, and the Space Between

Later, the house I had envisioned in my meditation became a real possibility. The challenge was never deciding to pursue it; the challenge was the uncertainty surrounding the process. The finalizing and signing of the necessary paperwork was taking much longer than anticipated, and the sellers had already extended the closing date twice. Each delay brought new questions and pressure. I worried constantly: Would this go through? Could I manage the timeline and all the logistics? What if it didn't close at all? It was impossible to control what others would do, and I realized that my anxiety and attachment were only adding stress without changing the outcome. I made a conscious decision to focus on what I could control and release what I could not. I told myself that if this house was meant to be, it would close, and if it was not, another opportunity would appear that aligned with my needs.

Making that choice to surrender was difficult. I had to acknowledge that I could not guarantee timing, cooperation from others, or the sequence of events. I had to accept that delays and obstacles were part of the process, not a reflection of my abilities or my worthiness. Letting go of attachment to the outcome allowed me to remain calm and clear-headed. I could take the actions that were mine to take, communicating, completing paperwork, and staying organized, without getting lost in worry or frustration over circumstances beyond my control. I realized that surrender is not passivity; it is an active choice to trust the process while doing everything you can on your side.

Through this experience, I learned that trust and patience are just as important as action. By letting go of my attachment to the timing and outcome, I was able to stay focused on what mattered most and respond to challenges with clarity rather than fear. I also realized that outcomes rarely unfold exactly as planned, and that life often requires us to act decisively while remaining open to uncertainty. The house eventually closed, aligning with my needs and vision, but the greater lesson was in how I approached the process: with trust, presence, and the willingness to release control. This approach strengthened my confidence, my resilience, and my ability to navigate future uncertainties without being paralyzed by fear or doubt.

The Keys to Trust and Transformation

I now understand that in moments of uncertainty, surrender is a conscious strategy, not a resignation. It allows you to stay committed to your goals, take responsibility for what is yours to do, and release energy spent on outcomes you cannot control. When we act decisively within our circle of influence and let go of what is outside it, we open ourselves to solutions and opportunities that may not have been visible when we were attached to a specific result. The process taught me that trust, patience, and clarity in action are just as important as the outcome itself, and that the universe often requires us to release control in order to move forward effectively with the best plan for our exponential growth

During my son's hospital stays, I reduced my work hours to focus on his care. It terrified me because it was such a significant change. I questioned myself constantly: Was this the right move? Would I have enough money to cover our needs? How would it affect my career long term? Was I being careless with my future? What about my retirement, my security, my professional reputation? Society constantly whispers that taking time away from work to care for children is a risk, that stability is paramount, and that the future must be guaranteed. My mind circled through every "responsible" paradigm: if I step back now, will I be falling behind? Will I regret this choice later? And yet, through all the noise and pressure, my intuition, the quiet inner voice, nudged me forward. I chose to follow it. That choice allowed me to coach and work from home, aligning perfectly with my larger vision of working from anywhere and having the freedom to shape my schedule.

Opportunities and experiences appeared that I could not have planned. I realized that fear often signals the path to the most significant growth, and that the universe uses these catalytic moments to push us toward transformation when we are ready to act. I learned that no matter how secure a job may seem or how carefully we try to plan the future, life is never guaranteed. The only certainty is the present moment and the choices we make within it. By trusting myself and knowing that the universe always delivers, I created a path that supported my family, honored my values, and allowed me to grow in ways that no rigid plan could have anticipated.

There were days when grief, fear, and uncertainty threatened to overwhelm me. I had learned to survive by reacting, controlling, and overthinking. Over time, I began to pause, breathe, and observe. Even in the middle of chaos, I noticed the space between triggers and my responses. I began choosing differently, to respond instead of react. One evening, sitting quietly in my son's hospital room, I did not focus on monitors, charts, or answers. I noticed his breathing, the warmth of his hand, the care of the nurses, the presence of my parents, the generosity of friends, and the specialized support we had access to in our city. In that moment, everything was okay. Presence became my source of peace, clarity, and courage, even amidst uncertainty.

I have come to understand that life constantly offers us keys: courage, intuition, presence, surrender, and deliberate action. Each of these keys is available to us in every moment, and every moment requires us to choose. There is no wrong choice, only choices not fully embraced. Every action, every risk, every step forward moves us closer to the life we are meant to create. Presence gives awareness, courage gives the strength to act, intuition provides guidance, surrender allows flow, and deliberate action transforms vision into reality.

Ask yourself: When was the last time you paused without judgment? When have you ignored your intuition out of fear or logic? Where could trusting yourself, embracing uncertainty, and taking aligned action open a new door for you today? Each step, each decision, each leap into fear and discomfort is an invitation to grow, expand, and create a life aligned with your highest self. The universe does not make mistakes. It mirrors the energy you carry, responds to the frequency you hold, and provides opportunities that match your readiness. By choosing courage over comfort, trust over doubt, and action over hesitation, you become the creator of your reality, the architect of your life, and the steward of your energy.

Your life is shaped by the choices you make in every moment. Big, scary leaps are not obstacles. They are catalysts. Moments of fear are signals that transformation is available. Presence allows you to see clearly. Intuition guides you. Courage propels you forward. Surrender allows the flow of opportunity. Deliberate action turns vision into reality. Every choice matters, every step counts, and every leap into the unknown shapes the path to the life you are meant to live. This is the work of creating a life aligned with your growth, your vision, and your highest self, moment by moment, decision by decision, breath by breath, because there are no wrong keys.

Reflection Exercises

Take a journal and spend some time with the following prompts:

- Where am I holding onto fear instead of trusting myself?

- What small action can I take today to align with my growth?

- How can I notice and appreciate the support around me?

- Which choice will move me forward, even if it feels uncomfortable?

- How will I respond with presence, clarity, and courage in this moment?

Affirmations

I release control over what I cannot change and focus on what I can.

Every challenge I face strengthens my resilience and growth.

I choose courage over fear, and action over hesitation.

My energy shapes my reality, and I protect it wisely.

I am capable of navigating uncertainty with calm and purpose.

Gratitude anchors me, even in difficult moments.

CLOSING OF SECTION THREE

You are not here to survive. You are here to reclaim your energy, your focus, and your life. Every challenge, every setback, every moment of fear or doubt is an invitation to rise. When you take full responsibility for your energy, physical, emotional, mental, and spiritual, you shift everything. Obstacles become momentum. Setbacks become lessons. Fear becomes clarity. Presence becomes power.

Every trigger, every mirror, every challenge is a chance to see where your energy wavers and where growth is waiting. The universe doesn't punish you; it shows you exactly where your power is ready to be claimed. Every pause, every intentional act, every moment of gratitude compounds, reshaping not only your experiences but the person you are becoming. Your energy is your source, and how you choose to wield it determines the life you attract.

Life doesn't demand perfection; it demands awareness, deliberate choice, and the courage to act even when it's hard. You have the strength to rise beyond limits, to expand your resilience, and to step fully into alignment with your highest self. This is your reclamation. Take ownership. Commit to growth. Elevate your life.

The moment you choose clarity, focus, and intention, you move beyond survival into acceleration. You rise. You expand. You transform. Your power, your potential, your limitless life—claim it now.

SECTION FOUR
THANKFUL BY DESIGN: GRATITUDE AS THE GATEWAY TO YOUR EXTRAORDINARY LIFE

What if every mistake was a message? Every hardship, a guide? What if the breakdowns weren't failures but feedback, clues, course corrections from a universe that was never punishing you, only preparing you?

The universe is constantly repurposing your pain into power. You weren't falling behind. You were being forged. Every detour shapes your strength. Every setback reroutes you back to your power. Resilience isn't just survival. It's your launchpad. And the greatest superpower you hold? The way you choose to respond to life's challenges by embracing them and welcoming them with gratitude.

Gratitude is a magnetic current that can shift the entire trajectory of your life and quantum leap growth and change if you choose it. The more you tune into gratitude, even in the midst of your most difficult challenges, the more the universe responds in return. Appreciation is one of the most powerful frequencies because what you focus on expands and what you celebrate moment to moment multiplies exponentially. Gratitude is not passive. It's intentional and a magnetic force that aligns you with infinite possibilities when you choose it.

Gratitude doesn't erase hardship or pretend pain isn't real, but it provides perspective on what you can control and guides you back to joy, wholeness, and bliss, even in the midst of chaos.

Gratitude is the doorway, and when you walk through it intentionally, it transforms your life, elevates your energy, and opens the gateway to limitless possibilities. The universe responds to the vibrations you carry. The more grateful you are, the more it gifts you. Gratitude is the ultimate growth engine. The ultimate frequency, your ultimate superpower. Hardships will happen in life no matter what, so why not embrace them with gratitude? Tune in. Feel it. Live it. Become it.

CHAPTER 16
QUANTUM GROWTH THROUGH SURRENDER: GRIEF IN REAL TIME

"Change the way you look at things and the things you look at change." — Wayne Dyer

---

Between Hope and Heartbreak

They say the universe only gives you what you can handle. I have come to believe this deeply, yet I resented it at times. What parent can watch their child's chest rise and fall with the help of machines and not feel helpless? What parent can live in the space between hope and heartbreak, between the life they envisioned and the reality they are forced to navigate? I realized that handling these moments is not about being unbreakable. It is about confronting the raw, intense reality of the situation and finding the strength to continue.

Every disrupted plan, every sleepless night, every unanswered question was not meant to destroy me but to teach me how to navigate challenges with presence, gratitude, and resilience. Grief did not arrive only after loss; it arrived in the form of uncertainty, of waiting, of watching my child struggle while trying to hold myself together. I felt a deep, continuous grief for the milestones we were missing: first days of school, vacations, family dinners without hospital equipment and alarms. I was not grieving his presence; I was grieving the life I thought we would have. At the same time, I wrestled with guilt. How could I grieve when he was still here? How could I allow myself to feel the pain without feeling selfish? The answer I discovered was that grief and love can coexist.

Feeling the full weight of this reality does not diminish my care for my child; it strengthens it. Living through uncertainty and pain taught me to focus on what I could control: my presence, my energy, my choices. Fear narrows focus, while trust expands it. Each day in the hospital required me to make decisions with clarity, gratitude, and compassion, even when the outcomes were unknown. I learned that the most profound growth happens in these moments of intensity. It is not about avoiding pain or bypassing fear. It is about confronting reality fully, managing your energy, and choosing how to respond. The universe does not ask for perfection; it asks for engagement, awareness, and the willingness to rise despite circumstances that feel overwhelming. These months were not only about surviving. They were about discovering strength, resilience, and clarity I did not know I had.

The World Doesn't Stop

One afternoon, I stood by the hospital window and looked across the street at the adult hospital where I worked. Outside, people were walking, talking, and carrying on with their lives. In that moment, a sharp truth became clear: The world does not stop for our pain, and it never will. I realized I had a choice. I could keep resisting, clinging to the life I thought we were supposed to have, or I could accept the reality in front of me and move forward with it. That decision to stop resisting was the beginning of a profound shift in how I approached everything. Pain and grief are unavoidable; they come whether we give permission or not. What is optional is how we manage them. I understood that joy and grief can coexist.

Some nights, I cried until I was exhausted. Some mornings, I laughed until my stomach ached. Both experiences were real, and both mattered. The turning point came when I consciously surrendered. This did not mean giving up; it meant taking full responsibility for how I carried my pain. I could choose to remain bitter and disconnected, a victim of circumstance, or I could see grief as a signal to grow into a stronger, more capable version of myself. I chose growth, and that choice changed everything. I learned that life does not respond to effort or struggle. It responds to the energy we carry.

When I chose gratitude over bitterness, trust over fear, and presence over escape, my life began to rearrange itself around these choices. Gratitude became my guide. It helped me notice small, ordinary moments of meaning: his laughter during treatments, the sunlight coming through the window, the gift of another day together. Gratitude did not remove the pain, but it allowed me to live fully alongside it. As I shifted my energy, support appeared, resilience increased, and new opportunities emerged. This experience was not about survival alone. It was about growth, clarity, and the deliberate expansion of my life in real time.

Redefining Resilience

I have met other parents who worried that their children were not "keeping up," not graduating, not driving themselves, not meeting the milestones of their peers. I have been there too, weighed down by expectations and comparisons. But I have learned that the hardest barriers are not out in the world; they are the ones we build in our minds. Our children were not falling behind; they were growing in ways the world cannot measure. They were learning compassion, grit, adaptability, courage, and forms of wisdom that most people do not encounter until much later in life. And we, as parents, were not just enduring. We were transforming.

Resilience is not simply survival; it is freedom. It is the ability to release what we cannot control and to trust that we can meet whatever comes next. Grief taught me that healing is not about fixing what is broken; it is about learning to live fully even while carrying the weight of what hurts. Pain does not cancel joy. They coexist. In that coexistence, life becomes deeper, richer, and more honest. I laugh and cry in the same day. I honor both the beauty and the challenge. I walk with grief rather than resisting it. That choice does not make me weaker; it makes me whole. I carry grief not as proof of failure but as proof of love. And in that love, I found gratitude. In gratitude, I found resilience. In resilience, I found growth and the ability to move forward intentionally. The universe does not respond to what happens to me. It responds to the energy I choose to carry.

Every time I choose presence, gratitude, and love, I rise. This is my practice: to live not in resistance but in deliberate alignment with the energy I choose, to walk fully with grief, gratitude, and love, and through that conscious choice to move toward the extraordinary life waiting beyond surrender.

Reflection Exercises

Take a journal and spend some time with the following prompts:

- Identify a thought you've been carrying that feels heavy (fear, pain, doubt). Ask yourself: What is this thought broadcasting to the universe?

- Reframe it into a frequency of power. Example: "I'm losing everything." Frequency Shift: "Life is reshaping me into who I was meant to become."

- Write down three lessons your current or past grief has taught you about strength, love, or presence. Then ask: If grief were a mentor, what is it training me for?

- What dreams or expectations am I mourning, even if life continues?

- Have I given myself permission to feel this grief without guilt?

- Write down one thing you're grateful for that exists only because of your pain or challenge. Example: Because of hospital nights, I learned presence. Because of uncertainty, I discovered resilience. This rewires the brain to see pain as an activator of growth, not just a thief of joy.

Affirmations

I choose presence over fear,
gratitude over resistance.

My energy is my power, and the
universe mirrors it back to me.

Every breath is a choice.
Every choice is a rise.

I walk with grief, I walk with love, and
in that union, I expand limitlessly.

CHAPTER 17
THRIVING THROUGH TRIBULATIONS: FINDING PURPOSE AND STRENGTH, ESPECIALLY IN THE MIDST OF CHAOS

"The wound is the place where the Light enters you." — Rumi

The Space Between Fear and Strength

There is a sound I will never forget, not from the outside world, but from within me. It was the sound of my heart breaking so intensely that it consumed everything else. That was the day my life split into before and after. We were not prepared. No parent ever is. One moment, life was filled with ordinary responsibilities, emails, groceries, hockey, laundry, and the next, we were thrust into a world no one warns you about: hospital corridors, specialists, white coats, endless tests, and impossible choices. The fear was no longer about me; it was about my child and the realization that I could not fix the pain or make it go away. That day broke me, not all at once, but piece by piece. It began with subtle symptoms, small signs that reminded me how quickly life can change. Then came the pause, the silence before the doctor spoke, the weight of measured words. That moment drew a clear line between who I had been and who I was required to become. I did not have the choice to escape reality, but I did have the choice of how to meet it. I could collapse under fear, or I could rise, one decision at a time.

I learned that instinct matters, as the quiet inner voice often carries more truth than the noise around you. Strength is not dramatic; it is in the consistent choices to keep showing up. Resilience is built in the hardest moments; it is forged in challenge, not comfort. Even in the most difficult circumstances, I am not powerless. I can control my presence, my energy, and my willingness to continue. That pause, the doctor's words, changed me forever. It shattered my old version of myself but revealed a new, determined version I had not known existed. I realized that the illusions of control, perfection, or rule following could not keep my child safe. What remained was raw and terrifying: fear, anger, helplessness, and beneath it all, a love so intense it consumed me. That love became the force that guided every choice, every breath, and every action in the days that followed.

During this time, I witnessed a depth of grief, fear, and responsibility I had never known. There were days I cried alone, nights I screamed into pillows so no one could hear, hours I spent pleading with the universe for a positive outcome. I was broken in ways I could not have predicted. And yet, I also began to see and recognize resilience in action: the way nurses cared for my son, the quiet support of other parents in the hallway, the small signs of progress that brought clarity and reassurance. I realized that grief and growth can coexist, that presence, gratitude, and love are choices I can make even in the hardest moments, and that the universe responds to the energy I carry rather than the events themselves.

Through all of this, I learned the value of presence. I learned to pause, to notice the space between my triggers and my reactions, to respond instead of react. In the hospital, I would sit quietly, observing my child's breathing, the care of staff, and the generosity of friends, colleuagues and family. I noticed how much support existed even in moments that felt unbearable. Those observations allowed me to choose differently, to act intentionally, and to align with my highest priorities. Presence gave me clarity, courage, and the ability to make decisions from a grounded place rather than from fear or obligation.

I also learned to trust my intuition. Every time I followed that quiet inner voice, whether reducing work hours, leaving my marriage, or pursuing opportunities like the house, the doors that opened were aligned with my vision and growth. Fear often signals the path to significant transformation. The universe nudges us toward catalytic changes when we are ready, and taking the leap, even when it is uncomfortable, is necessary for expansion. Every challenge became a lesson in resilience, every difficult choice an opportunity to build confidence, strength, and trust in myself.

I have learned that we are far stronger than we give ourselves credit for. We can endure more, grow more, and achieve more than we often believe. Trusting that the universe has our best interests at heart, that every situation has a reason and that timing matters, allows us to make choices from clarity rather than fear. Strength, resilience, and growth are built in the decisions we make, the presence we cultivate, and the energy we choose to carry. Every challenge, every pause, every step forward has shaped the life I am living now, and every moment continues to teach me how to navigate uncertainty with courage, clarity, and trust.

I realized that in every single moment I had a choice. I could hold on to bitterness, anger, or defeat, or I could surrender, not by giving up, but by letting go of the illusion that I was ever in control and consciously choose how I would respond. This was the moment I began listening, not just to doctors, but to something deeper: my intuition, my inner wisdom, and the universe waiting for me to hear.

This chapter of my life began with difficulty and uncertainty, but those challenges revealed strength I didn't know I had and clarity I had not yet accessed. I stopped seeing challenges as obstacles or punishments. I began to see them as opportunities meant to expand me into the person I am becoming. The universe places these moments on our path to encourage growth and action, not to defeat us. Every difficulty, every change, every shift became a chance to rise higher. What was difficult did not destroy me; it gave me choice. The choice to meet life with resistance or with commitment. The choice to respond with fear or with confidence. I now know I will never be the same, not because I was broken, but because I chose to grow. I chose to see clearly. I chose to welcome the process instead of resisting it. This is what happens when we stop asking, "Why me?" and start saying, "I will handle this because I am always supported."

My Energy, My Power, My Response: A Life Lived Fully

There was a time I believed life happened to me. That every setback, every mistake, every disappointment was evidence that I wasn't enough, that I was failing. I measured my worth by outcomes I could not control and by approval I didn't even want. In the quiet moments, when blame and shame faded, I realized something important: What felt like punishment was actually guidance. Every difficulty, the guilt I carried, the plans that didn't work out, was instruction. Every time I thought I had failed, I was learning. Every time I felt lost, the universe was guiding me back to strength and clarity. I noticed that life responds to the energy I bring into it, not my words or intentions alone. When I reacted from fear, I felt trapped and depleted. When I responded with presence, clarity, and deliberate choice, the world shifted. Opportunities appeared, support arrived, and solutions unfolded in ways I could not have planned. Every moment became a crossroads. Every breakdown, setback, or challenge was a chance to decide not just how I felt, but how I acted. I could respond with fear, defensiveness, or doubt, or I could respond with focus, clarity, and energy. The universe reflects back whatever frequency I choose to carry.

There were nights I lay awake, exhausted by the demands of life, believing I had nothing left to give. Yet in those quiet moments, I realized something essential: Transformation comes from aligning with yourself and investing your energy intentionally. It's not about doing more but choosing wisely, being fully present, and responding with clarity and responsibility. Showing up as myself, making decisions with intention, and trusting my guidance became the foundation for my growth. I began to see that I am far stronger and more resilient than I had ever believed. I can handle far more than I imagined, and when I trust the universe, its timing, and my own ability to act, I am capable of navigating uncertainty, making difficult choices, and creating the life I want. Every decision, every step, every moment of presence is proof of strength, resilience, and growth.

Setbacks became opportunities to learn and grow. Wrong turns became new directions that led to clarity and insight. Every experience I labeled as a failure became feedback. I realized the universe was not punishing me; it was teaching me how to recognize and use my own power. Every challenge trained me to respond thoughtfully instead of reacting automatically, to act with strength instead of collapsing under pressure. I began to respond differently. I forgave more quickly, trusted more deeply, and released what I could not control. I invested my energy in what truly aligned with my values and vision. Over time, I saw life reflect abundance, clarity, and growth back to me. Every decision, every perceived mistake, became a message. Every detour offered guidance. The universe does not waste our pain; it provides lessons that, when applied, transform our energy and our results.

I recognized that life unfolded in alignment with the energy I carried. I was not at the mercy of circumstances, and I noticed where I had been giving my power away to what I could not control. I choose my frequency, and I choose my responses. The universe reflected the energy I brought, and so I asked myself where I was still holding back, where fear or habit kept me from stepping fully into my power. What would change if you approached every difficulty with focus and purpose? Freedom is the ability to choose, and power comes from taking full responsibility for yourself. You do not have to shrink or step back. You can rise in every decision, every response, and every moment you are aware of.

This is your energy, and this is your life. You can hold space for yourself and recognize that your power is always available to claim. Every choice you make is an opportunity to exercise it. Are you willing to take it?

Reflection Exercises

Take a journal and spend some time with the following prompts:

- You will forget. You will react. But you can always choose again, moment to moment. Realignment is never out of reach. Think of a recent moment when you reacted in a way that didn't serve you. What would choosing again look like right now?

- Recall a moment when you felt "cracked open." What did it take from you? What did it give you?

- What illusions about control or safety shattered for you, and what truths emerged in their place?

- Not everything unfolds on your schedule. Some delays protect you; some detours prepare you. Trust that life's timing serves your growth, even when it challenges your patience. Where in your life are you rushing an outcome instead of allowing it to unfold?

- Where, even in pain, did gratitude show up unexpectedly?

Affirmations

I honor the cracks, for they are the openings for light.

I am allowed to break and rebuild; both are sacred.

My strength is not in pretending; my strength is in presence.

I trust that even in the breaking, I am being rebuilt even stronger.

CHAPTER 18
EMBRACING GROWTH AS A CONSCIOUS CHOICE: CHANGE DOES NOT HAPPEN BY CHANCE

"We are what we repeatedly do. Excellence, then, is not an act, but a habit." — Aristotle

---

Love in the Silence of Fear

I will never forget those hospital days, the constant beeping of machines, the tangled tubes, the sterile smells, the endless movement of scrubs around my son's fragile state. Every detail is etched into my memory eternally. Every pause, every breath, every decision carried weight. But what truly reshaped me was not just the crisis itself, but the grace, love, and presence that appeared in the middle of it. In those moments, I realized that even when life is hardest, we are never truly powerless. Presence matters more than control. Compassion matters more than perfection. Showing up fully, without needing to fix or solve, can be transformative.

When my parents came, we didn't speak much. Words felt insufficient in the face of raw fear and grief. And yet, their presence alone, standing beside his bed, crying quietly, holding space, reminded me that love and support can be steady and unwavering, even when silence is all that can be offered. My sister brought food, and generous gestures of care were deeply grounding and came from all directions. In the midst of chaos, I noticed that love doesn't need to be loud or performative. It can be quiet, consistent, and profoundly felt.

The staff from the unit my son had been on before coming to ICU became an unexpected source of warmth and inspiration. They created a memory book for him, filling each page with glimpses of his personality, his quirks, his humor, the small things that made him uniquely himself. They didn't stop there. Understanding the intensity of the ICU environment, they coordinated a schedule to visit him on their breaks, ensuring he had a familiar, comforting presence throughout the day. Watching their dedication and thoughtfulness, I felt a quiet reassurance wash over me. Even amidst tubes, monitors, and uncertainty, their actions showed me that presence, commitment, and genuine care can transform even the most difficult moments into spaces of connection, hope, and resilience. One special physician returned after her shift just to sit with him and read. She offered her time and attention without any expectation. These acts of commitment left an everlasting impact on me and my family, and to this day, I remember how grateful we were to have them and how their support meant the world.

During that time, I realized that fear, grief, and uncertainty are inevitable, but how we respond is a choice. I had a choice every day: to cling to anger, resentment, or helplessness, or to step into clarity, presence, and responsibility for my own energy. I could resist the reality around me or I could engage fully with it, without trying to control what I could not. This understanding reshaped the way I approached every decision and every interaction. I stopped asking "Why me?" and began asking, "What can I learn here? How can I rise here?"

I also learned that we are far stronger than we give ourselves credit for. I had no idea that I could endure sleepless nights, advocate fiercely, and maintain presence while sitting beside my child in critical condition. I discovered a resilience I hadn't known existed. And I realized that growth often comes in the moments that scare us most, when the universe nudges us to take action, even when everything about the situation is uncertain. Every step I took in trust, every small decision to show up, aligned me with opportunities and insights I could never have planned.

One of the clearest lessons was the power of surrender. There were situations I could not control: test results, procedures, timelines, and even family dynamics. Instead of resisting, I began to release attachment to outcomes I could not influence. I trusted that I was being taken care of, that there was a reason and divine timing for everything, and that the universe had my best interests at heart. This mindset did not make the fear disappear, but it gave me clarity and strength to act from a place of presence rather than panic.

Gratitude became a lifeline. Even amid the hardest moments, I noticed the small acts of care: a nurse holding a hand, a technician offering a reassuring word, the warmth of my family's presence. These moments reminded me that love and connection are constants, even in the face of uncertainty. I began to see that pain and gratitude can coexist, and that acknowledging both allows life to expand rather than contract. I could meet grief, fear, and uncertainty not as obstacles, but as invitations to practice my own courage, clarity, and growth.

Rising Through Presence and the Grace of Others

From that time, I carry three truths that guide me every single day. First, surrender creates space for clarity and opportunity. When I let go of attachment to outcomes I cannot control, I noticed possibilities I might have otherwise missed. Second, connection is essential. Even small gestures, a hand held, a tear shared, a kind word, provide stability and remind us we are not alone. Third, love is infinite and enduring. The care we give, and the care we witness, resonates far beyond the immediate moment. It shapes us, strengthens us, and reminds us of the potential within ourselves to respond with grace, even in the hardest circumstances.

Every challenge I faced during that time became an opportunity to practice presence, awareness, and intentional action. I learned that life does not respond to effort alone, but to the energy we bring, to the choices we make, and to the mindset we cultivate. Fear and grief are inevitable, but they do not define us. Our responses do. And when we choose clarity, presence, and intentionality, life reflects it back to us in ways that expand our resilience, growth, and capacity for love.

Through that period, I discovered that I am stronger and more capable than I ever allowed myself to believe. I learned that I can endure, adapt, and respond with wisdom and compassion, even when circumstances are beyond my control. I realized that every challenge, every difficult choice, and every moment of uncertainty is an opportunity to rise into the person I am meant to become. And I know now, with absolute certainty, that the universe supports us when we act with integrity, presence, and trust, and that there is always a reason and divine timing for every experience.

I left the ICU forever changed. Not just because my son survived, but because I witnessed the depth of human care and support in ways that reshaped how I see the world. Nurses, staff, family, and friends consistently went beyond their duties, taking the time to hold his hand, read to him, and acknowledge him as a person, not just a patient. My parents, family, and friends were present, helping with my other children and providing support in all forms. Friends offered rides, meals, and practical help that made it possible for me to focus on my son. Even small gestures, a meal delivered, a note of encouragement, a quiet check-in, reminded me that support exists all around us when we are open to receiving it. These experiences showed me that presence, care, and attention are powerful forms of love and support, and that we are never truly alone, even in the most difficult moments.

Even in life's hardest moments, transformation is possible. Every act of support, every gesture of care, every moment of presence, whether offered by others or cultivated within ourselves, is fuel for resilience, growth and strength. Every difficulty holds the potential for exponential growth, and every conscious choice propels us forward faster than we ever imagined.

I have learned that life's gifts are often quiet, waiting for us to notice them. When I pause, I see the support that has always been around me, the strength I didn't know I carried. I wonder, have you paused lately to see what is holding you up? Have you allowed yourself to truly receive it?

There were moments when I acted without awareness, moving through life on autopilot, thinking progress was measured by doing more, pushing harder. And yet, the real breakthroughs came when I slowed, when I chose to act with intention. Ask yourself, where could your awareness create your next breakthrough? Where might a small shift in focus open a path you hadn't seen before?

I have felt fear and doubt try to make me small, to keep me from stepping fully into my power. And each time I refused to shrink, life expanded in ways I could not have predicted. I wonder what part of yourself have you been holding back? What might happen if you allowed yourself to rise fully, without apology, without hesitation?

Every moment offers the same choice I face: to stay stuck in reaction, or to step forward with clarity and purpose. Awareness, presence, deliberate action, they are not just ideas, they are game changers. How will you use them today? How will you honor the power and gifts already within you, and the support already surrounding you, to create a life that reflects your highest potential?

Reflection Exercises

Take a journal and spend some time with the following prompts:

- Who has offered support or presence to you, and how did it impact your ability to respond to challenges?

- How can you show up for others without feeling the need to control or solve outcomes?

- What fears might you release by trusting the support and timing present in your life?

- How might focusing on gratitude for practical support, care, and presence shift your energy and resilience?

Affirmations

I notice and appreciate the small blessings in every moment.

Gratitude anchors me in strength, presence, and possibility.

Every choice I make, every action I take, contributes to my growth and impact.

I claim full responsibility for my energy, my choices, and my life.

I step fully into my power, even in the hardest moments.

CHAPTER 19
RECLAIM YOUR POWER, REWRITE YOUR STORY, RISE INTO LIMITLESSNESS

"The more you practice the art of thankfulness,
the more you have to be thankful for."
— Norman Vincent Peale

The Night That Changed Everything

There are moments in life that pause time. Moments that don't just happen, they reach inside of you, shift the ground beneath your feet, and rearrange something at the core of your being eternally. You recognize in those moments, that you are forever changed and will never be the same.

One of those moments for me was the night I received the call that my son had been rushed to the hospital by ambulance, requesting that I come to the hospital to meet the ambulance there.

The seconds after the phone rang were surreal. My chest tightened so sharply that I thought my heart stopped beating. My breath came in short, uneven gasps and my mind was blank except for one repeating thought: *Will he be okay this time?*

The drive to the hospital was a blur. I could not remember the turns I took, even though it was the exact route I took to go to the adult hospital I worked at just next door. The steering wheel beneath my hands, the lights flashing by, it was as though my body moved without me, guided by some instinctual force of nature, carrying me forward while my mind floated elsewhere, suspended outside of my body and somewhere between panic and disbelief.

When I arrived, chaos met me immediately. The trauma room pulsed with urgency: machines beeped in sharp, relentless rhythms, voices floated everywhere with commands, scrubs moved faster than I could follow, reacting instinctively to what my brain struggled to process. I had been in rooms like this before, as a healthcare professional trained to assess, act, and intervene, but this time, it was very different. I wasn't in control. I wasn't the provider. I was a mother, powerless in the face of circumstances

I could not influence. And for the first time in my life, I understood what it truly meant to feel helpless.

I froze, unable to speak, unable to move. Fear gripped me with a force that felt physical, like it had replaced my entire body and paralyzed me. Then, a woman I didn't know approached me. She wasn't in scrubs, but she was part of the team. She moved slowly, deliberately, and with calm intent.

"Is there anything I can do for you?" she asked.

I tried to answer. No words came.

"I can hold your hand, if you want," she said.

I nodded. Her hand slid into mine, warm, steady, unshakable. She didn't try to distract me, didn't offer promises she couldn't keep, didn't soften the storm around me. She simply was. Present, grounded and human.

For the first time that night, I felt like I was not alone.

Moments later, another person entered, a young resident I knew from the adult hospital I worked at. He noticed me, a crumbling version of myself standing there, and his eyes found mine. In that instant, I broke down and started crying.

The tears came without warning. Shame followed, the professional in me undone, exposed, trembling before a colleague. He was quiet and very much a pivotal part of the decision making for the next steps in my son's care that night. The only words he spoke were, "I'm so sorry, Angèle," but his presence and compassion were so deep that, to this day, those words echo in my soul and I am forever grateful. He simply held space for me in a compassionate and loving way while he performed his medical duties.

And in that silence, I realized something profound: Sometimes the essence of support, of strength, of real resilience, is not in what you do. It is in what you allow others to do for you as the receiver. Presence. Witnessing. Showing up fully without expectation or solutions. That is what carried me in that moment when I couldn't carry myself.

When the chaos settled and my body finally exhaled, I felt the residue of that night, not as memory, but as energy. The way the resident held space for me. The warmth of the hand that held mine. Those gestures were more than comfort; they were frequencies, steady, grounded, compassionate. They spoke a language beyond words, one my nervous system understood before my mind could translate.

That experience shifted something fundamental in me. I realized resilience isn't about pushing through; it's about allowing energy to move through. It's not about hardening, it's about expanding our capacity to stay open, even when everything inside us wants to shut down.

True empowerment isn't found in resistance. It's found in awareness in choosing peace over protection, presence over performance, and love over fear.

That night taught me that the most powerful people aren't the ones who never fall apart. They're the ones who know how to return to themselves, gently, honestly, and whole.

Resilience, I realized, isn't built on action alone. It isn't measured by effort or grit. It is alignment. It is learning to shift into higher states of being, even when fear, chaos, or uncertainty take over.

Resilience is energy in motion. Supported by presence, by love, by gratitude, by connection. These are frequencies. They ripple outward. They transform what they touch. They change everything around them.

Every thought, every choice, every gesture carries energy. And the universe responds. That night, the universe spoke through human hands and hearts. It reminded me I am never alone, even in my darkest hour.

Frequency of Strength: Transforming Challenge into Conscious Growth

And in that frequency, I also discovered active gratitude. Choosing to notice the small, stabilizing moments, even while the storm is raging. Choosing to see the good that is happening in real time: a hand to hold, steady eyes, a breath that reminds you you are alive. Gratitude is a frequency itself, anchoring and expanding you, reminding you that you can receive, and that rising is possible even when you can't breathe and withstand yet another heartbreak.

Even when everything outside is chaos, we always have choice. We may not choose the events, the storms, or the suffering, but we choose how we respond. Moment by moment, thought by thought, action by action.

Choosing fear doesn't make life stop. Choosing presence, awareness, love, or gratitude creates ripples that shape the world around you. Choosing awareness over autopilot, connection over isolation, trust over panic: These are the choices that allow us to rise again and again, even through the storm.

I carried a vow out of that trauma room: to live consciously, aware of the energy I bring into every space, every relationship, and into my own life. I committed to aligning myself with actions, thoughts, and interactions that expand rather than contract me. This awareness is not passive; it is a daily practice of choosing presence and energy in every moment.

Perseverance is not simply enduring life's challenges. True perseverance is rising through them consciously, moment by moment, recognizing that each difficulty is an opportunity to grow, to expand, and to strengthen the core of who you are. Every challenge is a test of focus, resilience, and deliberate choice. Growth is not accidental; it is cultivated through awareness, discipline, and conscious engagement with life.

Gratitude anchors this process. It grounds us in the present, highlights what is working, and ensures that even amidst chaos, we notice what is constructive, true, and supportive. The universe reflects the energy we carry. It responds not to words but to the vibration of our focus, our intention, and our presence. Protect your energy. Honor it. Expand it. The quality of your life is directly proportional to the energy you cultivate, maintain, and release. When you operate from clarity, alignment, and strength, your life begins to mirror the highest version of yourself.

This chapter is not solely about a night in a hospital. It is about the lessons embedded in presence, trust, and conscious surrender. It is about reclaiming the power to allow support, to receive care, and to rise intentionally into the strength that has always been within you. Life becomes a deliberate practice when you recognize that you are the creator of your energy and determine the outcomes.

Gratitude is the foundation of conscious living. It anchors your attention in what is working, what is supportive, and what is true. The practice of gratitude trains your awareness to notice the forces that elevate you, strengthens your resilience, and empowers your decisions. When you tune into this frequency consistently, it becomes a compass guiding you to live fully, act intentionally, and design a life defined by clarity, alignment, limitless possibilities and extraordinary results.

Reflection Exercises

Take a journal and spend some time with the following prompts:

- Who in your life has shown up for you unexpectedly, and how did it shape your experience?

- How can you offer presence to others without needing to fix or control?

- What fears could you release if you fully surrendered to the grace of support around you?

- How might cultivating gratitude for the unseen helpers in your life shift your energy and resilience?

- What small moments of presence can you notice, even when everything feels uncertain?

- How can you use gratitude to shift your energy in real time?

- Where can you stop resisting life and start observing its messages instead?

- How would your life change if you trusted that your energy is magnetic and the universe is responding to it?

Affirmations

I am never truly alone. Love and support flow to me through seen and unseen hands. I surrender, I trust, and I receive the grace the universe delivers through others. My heart is open, my soul is resilient, and I am held.

CHAPTER 20
THE MAGNETIC POWER OF GRATITUDE

"When you arise in the morning, think of what a precious privilege it is to be alive—to breathe, to think, to enjoy, to love." — Marcus Aurelius

---

I'll never forget that call; it carried a heaviness I had grown all too familiar with. The voice on the other end was calm but heavy, and in a few words, my world blurred: My oldest son had been transferred to the ICU. My body acted before my mind could process. I grabbed my keys and ran to the car, tears streaming, breath coming in uneven gasps. The drive was tense and urgent, my thoughts consumed by fear and disbelief.

When I arrived at the hospital, the halls were bright, sterile, and painfully familiar. I had been here many times before and today, I was not in control. I was a mother, scared, exposed, and raw, trying to hold myself together while every part of me wanted to break. On my way to the ICU, I ran into a physician who had cared for my son over the years, but this time it was very different. She looked at me with a soft smile, and as tears rolled down my cheeks, she hugged me tightly. It's amazing how such a small gesture could transcend words and spark deep gratitude, bringing me a sense of comfort and relief in overwhelming darkness. That moment reminded me that you are never truly alone and shaped my perspective going forward. I realized that, even when life doesn't always go as planned, it would be okay if I consciously chose it to be. Though I hadn't elected this hardship for my family, I figured I could fall into one of two categories: I could either choose to live life by default, as though life was happening to me, and fall victim to my circumstances or I could live by design and accept that life is always happening for me and embrace the transformative power. And so, I began my Gratitude Campaign, making the conscious decision of embracing gratitude in every single thing, person, and event that crossed my path. Living life fully, as though it was my last day on earth, by design and in full appreciation of the NOW.

Sitting beside my son's bed, surrounded by

machines beeping and humming, I felt panic rise. The fluorescent lights reflected off the polished floor, harsh and unrelenting. I noticed how quickly my mind spun toward worst-case scenarios, how easily fear can consume you if you let it. But then I noticed something else: One thought, a single conscious choice, could shift my inner state completely. I could not control the medical outcome. I could not dictate the hours ahead. But I could choose my perspective. I could choose whether to focus on fear or on gratitude for what was still present: the doctors working tirelessly, the nurses moving with purpose and care, the faint rise and fall of my son's chest, evidence of life persisting against all odds.

That choice became my lifeline. It was what I now call living by design: Consciously deciding how to meet life moment by moment. It wasn't pretending that the pain didn't exist. It was refusing to let fear dominate, refusing to let the difficulty define the totality of the experience.

I practiced gratitude every day, even when it felt impossible. I focused on my son's breathing, the care of nurses and doctors, the small acts of support around me. Each choice to notice and acknowledge shifted me from fear to clarity.

I did not wait for life to get easier. I chose to engage

fully with what was present. Every moment I responded with awareness and gratitude, I reclaimed my energy, steadied my mind, and strengthened my ability to act intentionally.

Gratitude became my anchor. It gave me clarity, resilience, and the power to make deliberate choices, even in the hardest moments. Every conscious decision shaped my reality. I learned that I am not at the mercy of circumstances. I am responsible for my energy, my focus, and my response.

I rise through every challenge. I act with clarity. I choose presence. I reclaim my power.

Over the years, working with cancer patients in the hospital, I observed that consistent truth. Families and patients who practiced gratitude, even amidst heartbreak, carry a different energy. They do not deny their pain; they faced it directly while remaining open to connection and moments of care received. That choice transformed fear into faith, helplessness into empowerment, and despair into resilience. I remember one patient's spouse who, even in the depth of grief, took a moment to express gratitude for the care provided, just a few hours after his passing. That simple act left a lasting impression on me and reinforced a powerful lesson: The impact of a moment is defined not by the circumstances, but by how we choose to respond. Every day in the hospital reaffirmed that energy matters. Every thought, choice, and emotion carries weight. Operating from fear, anger, or resentment magnifies distress, while choosing gratitude, even in the hardest moments, creates alignment, opens the door to possibility, and supports healing for everyone involved.

During those long hours at the bedside, I realized that life will happen whether we resist it or not. Resisting fear, trying to control outcomes, or wishing things were different only drains energy. Change begins the moment you decide to take full responsibility for your life. It begins when you stop waiting for circumstances to improve and make the conscious choice to take control. It happens when you understand that you are not a bystander. You are the one who decides what comes next.

I didn't learn this from a classroom or a motivational event. I learned it in one of the hardest places imaginable, a hospital room.

That journey taught me that gratitude is not just a concept. It's real power. It's a decision to direct your focus toward what supports you rather than what drains you. It reshapes the way you think, feel, and act. It transforms fear into steadiness and pain into growth. True healing begins when we shift our inner state, not when the situation changes.

Who you become depends on what you choose to believe. When you live with intention, you stop reacting to what happens and begin creating the life you want. Even in the hardest moments, you have the ability to stand up, move forward, and redefine what's possible for you.

That awareness changed me forever. It changed the way I held space for my son, for my family, and for myself. I stopped reacting and began choosing. I anchored my energy even when everything around me felt unstable. And in that choice, I discovered freedom. In that freedom, I discovered the power to rise. Not by force, but by frequency. Not by struggle, but by alignment. Not by control, but by presence.

You were never meant to shrink. You were meant to rise, fully, intentionally, energetically alive. Gratitude is your access point. Your internal compass. Your frequency of freedom. When you embody it, life responds. Opportunities, alignment, and joy are drawn to your energy. Even in waiting, even in pain, even in uncertainty, you are becoming, being reshaped and supported.

Hardships are universal, but how you choose to face them defines you. Everyone experiences challenges, loss, and uncertainty. The difference lies in what you choose to focus on. Gratitude doesn't ignore pain; it gives you the power to move through it with strength and clarity.

Gratitude is a mindset. It's the decision to focus on what's working instead of what's missing, to see value where others see limitations. It's not about pretending life is perfect. It's about choosing to take ownership of your perspective, even when things are hard.

It's about noticing what's still right, the person who shows up for you, the breath that keeps you steady, the meal that reminds you that you're cared for. These small acknowledgments don't erase the pain, but they shift your focus toward what gives you stability and purpose.

Gratitude is the bridge between who you've been and who you are becoming. It grounds you in the present while expanding you into your highest potential. When you choose gratitude, you no longer move through life unconsciously, you move with awareness, intention, and purpose. You stop fighting against what is and begin to flow with it, trusting that every moment is part of your evolution.

You are no longer defined by your past or your pain. You are defined by the energy you choose right now. Every thought, every word, every action sends a ripple into your reality. When you embody gratitude, you raise your vibration, attract aligned opportunities, and create from a place of clarity and truth.

This is your invitation to live consciously, to wake up each day knowing that you are powerful beyond measure, that your energy is your creation tool, and that everything you experience is guiding you closer to your purpose.

Live with awareness. Lead with gratitude. Align with your highest frequency. The life you've imagined is already waiting for you, it begins the moment you decide to live in alignment with who you truly are, limitless and unstoppable.

Gratitude is the highest frequency, the vibration of freedom and limitless power. When you align with it, the universe matches your energy, reflecting back abundance, clarity, and expansion. Tune in fully, and let gratitude lead you home to your true power.

Reflection Exercises

Take a journal and spend some time with the following prompts:

- What is one small detail I often overlook that I can appreciate today?

- Who in my life has supported me quietly, and how can I acknowledge them?

- Which challenges or hardships have taught me lessons I am grateful for?

- What strengths have I discovered in myself through difficult moments?

- How has my perspective shifted when I focus on what is present rather than what is missing?

Affirmations

♡

Gratitude recalibrates my energy
to the frequency of abundance.
I am aligned with the vibration
of appreciation—where miracles
manifest easily.

My gratitude codes my reality
for expansion and ease.

I am thankful for every frequency
shift that elevates my life.

I give thanks in advance for
all that's unfolding perfectly.

Gratitude transforms my energy, and
my energy transforms my world.

Through gratitude, I create
quantum growth in every area of
my life.

CLOSING OF SECTION 4

You have come full circle. Every challenge, every breakthrough, every quiet moment of awakening has led you here, to this truth: *you are the creator of your energy, your experience, your life*. Gratitude is not just a practice; it's a way of being. It's the bridge between who you were and who you are becoming, a conscious, empowered, and limitless creator.

When you live with gratitude, you rise beyond reaction and into intention. You stop seeking external validation because you realize everything you've ever needed has always existed within you. You no longer wait for life to change before you feel peace; you choose peace and watch life rearrange itself to meet you there. Gratitude becomes your compass, your calibration point, your return to truth.

The universe has been guiding you all along through the lessons, the redirections, the moments that felt like endings but were actually beginnings. Every experience has been refining your alignment, strengthening your trust, and preparing you to live from expansion, not contraction.

Now, you know: freedom isn't something you chase; it's something you remember. Power isn't something you find; it's something you embody. Gratitude is the key that unlocks it all.

So, as you close these pages, carry this truth forward:

Live intentionally. Love expansively, especially when it's hard and lead your life with gratitude.

Every sunrise, every breath, every moment is an invitation to return, again and again, to your truth, your power, and your infinite wisdom and limitless potential.

You are thankful by design.
You are powerful by choice.
And you are limitless by nature.

♡

AUTHOR'S NOTE

I was born with a vision of a universe radiant, abundant, and limitless. A world where everyone thrives, where no one is forgotten, where worth is not ranked by race, gender, religion, status, or circumstance. In this vision, love was the currency of power, and life flowed with ease. Beings of all kinds, humans and animals, lived in harmony, moving together in a rhythm of oneness. Talents, gifts, and resources were shared freely. There was no competition, no scarcity, no hierarchy of value.

Again and again, this vision returned to me as a vivid dream so real it felt like an inner calling. Abundance was effortless, connection was natural, and unity was the law of existence. As a child, I felt it in every fiber of my being. I knew heaven on earth wasn't fantasy and that everyone was meant to live an extraordinary life.

But then reality settled in. I remember sitting cross-legged on the living room floor at six years old, watching commercials that made my stomach ache; children in Africa, their faces swarmed with flies, bellies bloated from hunger, eyes hollow with despair. I couldn't understand it. I begged my parents to send our leftovers in an envelope, anything to help. They explained gently that it wasn't that simple, that the world's problems were bigger than what we could fix sometimes. But all I knew was that the pain in my heart was real: Why can't we just do something? Why can't we just fix it?

That's when I made a quiet decision: That power lived outside of me, that change was someone else's responsibility, that one person could never possibly make a world of difference. As I grew older, I learned contrast. I learned the stories we're all taught: life is hard, survival is the goal, worth must be earned, and power belongs only to the few. Slowly, like so many of us, I began to shrink. I buried my vision under fear, doubt, and conformity.

Maybe you've felt it too, the ache of remembering a truth. That paralyzing sense that you're too small, too much of a dreamer, asking for too much, demanding more than life is willing to give. The whisper of your ego: *Who are you to believe in more? Who are you to think you can change the world? You are too loud, too much.*

And yet, despite all of it, the vision lives and pulses inside of you, waiting for the truth to be remembered. It surfaces in moments of presence, of connection, of sudden clarity when your heart remembers what your mind has tried to bury. The vision waits. Patiently. Urgently. For you to remember. For you to rise.

That call to rise is not for someday, not when it's convenient, not when the world finally grants you permission. The call is for *NOW*. Especially now. In a world of polarities, division, pain, war, and global crisis, your vision is not too small. It is absolutely necessary. Your rising is not optional; it's the answer we've been waiting for.

Through spiritual awakening and deep inner work, I've come to see that what the world most needs sometimes is not grand gestures or distant saviors: It is us. It is how we show up, how we live, how we love, how we move through the ordinary moments of our lives. Change begins with the energy we carry, in the quiet spaces of our hearts, in the generosity we cultivate, in the integrity we embody when no one is watching.

We are not here to fix the world for anyone else. We are not here to carry the weight of their choices or decide their path. We are here to claim the full measure of our own power, the frequency we carry, the light we shine, the love we cultivate. Harmony begins within. The world mirrors what we radiate. Every thought we hold, every word we speak, every action we take sends ripples across reality, echoes that stretch farther than we will ever see, shaping lives, shaping hearts, shaping futures.

You are never too small to make a difference. You are not powerless. You are energy. You are vibration. You are the Frequency. You are the answer the world needs at the moment.

The question is not whether you're powerful enough; it's what you will do with that power. Because every single one of us is already impacting the collective. Every thought you nurture, every word you speak, everything you choose to engage in, every choice you make sends ripples outward. You are shaping the world whether you acknowledge it or not. The only question is: what kind of world are you creating?

When you reclaim your energy, you give permission to others to reclaim theirs. This is how worlds change, not by waiting, not by hoping, not by asking, but by remembering who you are and always have been and living in the higher vibrations of love, joy, and gratitude.

The truth is very simple: No one's coming to save us.

No system, no leader, no perfect timing. The answer has always been inside of you. We are the revolution. We are the vision remembered. We are the power we've been waiting for. The vision I carried as a child was never a fantasy. It was a blueprint, a collective awakening. It is possible. It is real. It is waiting, and it all begins with you. It begins with us. Not someday. Not later. Not when the world is ready. It begins now. This is your call. This is your choice. Rise. Remember. Reclaim your power. Ignite the ripple that becomes a wave, the wave that becomes a movement, the movement that becomes our future. The world cannot afford to wait, and neither can you. The Frequency Effect is here. It's now. In this breath. In this choice. Right now, the power is yours.

And hear this too: We are stronger together. When we rise as a collective, mountains move, Timelines shift, Generations heal, Futures are rewritten.

So I *challenge* you:

What legacy are you living right now?

What frequency are you sending into your family, your community, your world?

What kind of human do you want to be remembered as when you leave? Your ripple begins here. Your wave begins now. The time is yours. The world is yours and waiting for your frequency: unafraid, unstoppable, luminous.

Infinite Blessings your way today, and always.

Angèle xo

ABOUT THE AUTHOR

Angèle Lamothe is a transformational speaker, empowerment coach, TEDx speaker, #1 bestselling author, and high-vibrational leader who helps people reclaim their energy, master their mindset, and create extraordinary lives. With a degree in Psychology, a Master's in Health Sciences, and training in both energy medicine and leadership, she fuses science and soul to equip people with the tools to thrive in even the toughest moments.

Her resilience was born from deeply personal, life-changing challenges with her child, moments that could have broken her, but instead ignited her philosophy that energy and mindset are the keys to transformation. By choosing her energy in the hardest seasons, she discovered how to turn pain into power, adversity into acceleration, and obstacles into opportunities.

Today, she guides others to do the same, helping driven individuals turn challenges into quantum leaps and create ripple effects of transformation in their families, communities, and the world.

Her mission is simple yet profound: to help you reclaim your energy, master your mindset, and design a life that is extraordinary in every sense. Angèle doesn't just inspire. She transforms. For those ready to stop surviving and start thriving, her work is a catalyst for quantum leaps, breakthroughs, and lasting change.

Website: angelelamothecoaching.com

Email: angelelamothecoaching@gmail.com

thank you

Dear Reader,

You made it! Thanks for sticking with me through these pages. I hope they brought you insights and sparks of inspiration. Sharing these stories and lessons has been an incredible journey, and it means so much that you chose to be a part of it too.

Now, if I could ask a quick favor: If you enjoyed the book, would you kindly leave a positive review on Amazon or Goodreads? It would truly make my day, and it's one of the best ways to help others find this book and maybe spark their own adventures. Your review might just be the encouragement someone else needs to give them permission to break from routine and empower them to make the change they need.

With deepest gratitude,

Angèle xo

MY GIFT TO YOU

I am so glad you're here!

As my gift to you, enjoy FREE access to the audiobook
The Frequency Effect!

Simply scan the QR code below or visit
angelelamothecoaching.com to find out when
it will be available for free download.

www.ingramcontent.com/pod-product-compliance
Lightning Source LLC
Chambersburg PA
CBHW070059030426
42335CB00016B/1941